Smart at Heart

smart at
HEART

a holistic 10-step approach to preventing
and healing heart disease for women

Malissa Wood, MD,
and Dimity McDowell

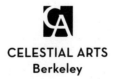

CELESTIAL ARTS
Berkeley

To the Corrigan-Minehan family, whose generosity and vision led to the founding of HAPPY Heart. Thank you also to the participants and staff of HAPPY Heart for your unending cooperation, assistance, and enthusiasm.

Published in the United States by Celestial Arts, an imprint of the Crown Publishing Group, a division of Random House, Inc., New York.
www.crownpublishing.com
www.tenspeed.com

Celestial Arts and the Celestial Arts colophon are registered trademarks of Random House, Inc.

Illustration on page 15 copyright © Athanasia Nomikou/Shutterstock.com

Library of Congress Cataloging-in-Publication Data
Wood, Malissa.
  Smart at heart : a holistic 10-step approach to preventing and healing heart disease for women / Malissa Wood and Dimity McDowell. — 1st ed.
    p. cm.
  Summary: "A mind-body program to build a strong, healthy, and happy heart, for women at risk for or diagnosed with heart disease"—Provided by publisher.
  Includes bibliographical references and index.
  1. Heart—Diseases—Alternative treatment. 2. Holistic medicine. 3. Women—Health and hygiene. 4. Heart—Diseases I. McDowell, Dimity. II. Title.
  RC684.A48W66 2011
  616.1'06—dc23

                    2011036470

ISBN 978-1-58761-278-7
eISBN 978-1-58761-281-7

Printed in the United States of America

Cover design by Betsy Stromberg
Interior design by Colleen Cain

10 9 8 7 6 5 4 3 2 1

First Edition

CONTENTS

INTRODUCTION

The year 2006 wasn't a great one for me. In June, I lost my nephew in a tragic accident. In October, my mother died of complications from a stroke. In addition, my eleven-year-old son, one of my four children, was diagnosed with autism spectrum disorder. I also made the tough decision to finalize my divorce. My ex-husband and I realized that despite our friendship and mutual commitment to raising our children, we could not bridge the gap in our friendship that had formed over time. All that tough news was on top of the whopper I received in December 2006: I had breast cancer. I almost couldn't believe it; I was a healthy forty-three-year-old woman who had run four marathons and adhered to a primarily vegetarian diet for most of my adult life. And now I had a potentially fatal disease.

While I was recovering from surgery and waiting to find out whether or not the cancer had spread to my lymph nodes, Kelly, a twenty-year survivor of ovarian cancer and a friend of a friend, came to see me. The morning of her visit, she brought me coffee and muffins. More importantly, she brought me hope. She told me that a cancer diagnosis was in fact an opportunity. With a fresh, invigorated perspective, her cancer gave her the chance to appreciate the beauty around her, reassess how she spent her time, and focus on being healthy for the rest of her life. "Crisis can equal opportunity," she told me as we sat on the sofa drinking coffee, me cozily wrapped in my favorite pink fluffy robe. She reached out and held my hand as tears rolled down both our cheeks. She told me I would emerge from this experience transformed, stronger, and more resilient than ever.

Fortunately, the cancer hadn't spread, but I realized I needed to pay attention to her important message. Earlier in 2006, I had also laid the foundation for a study I called HAPPY Heart. Medical studies are often known by an acronym, a word that describes what the study does using most or all of the first letters of the study's title; I wanted to come up with something that would reflect healthy habits and healthy, happy hearts. *HAPPY* stands for Heart Awareness and Primary Prevention in Your neighborhood. As I was washing dishes one night, the expanded title just popped into my head, and so I had the first, and perhaps hardest, step completed: getting started.

In many ways, HAPPY Heart was the natural progression for my somewhat untraditional career path as an academic cardiologist. A little history: because my then-husband had a military payback obligation in San Antonio, my first job as a physician was in Texas, which was far away, both physically and culturally, from Boston, where I had completed my internship, residency, and fellowship. In my practice in Texas, I took care of many young women who already had two strikes against them when it came to cardiovascular disease: a genetic history of heart disease and unhealthy lifestyles. Plus they had very little access to resources to help change their lives. I did my best to provide the clinical care, access to information, and support necessary to get the women motivated. I spent time with each patient, describing the steps they needed to take to improve their health. I referred them to a dietitian and got them started in safe, practical exercise programs. I knew that the women had the power within themselves to make huge life changes; they just needed a gentle push and the right kind of information.

As I saw patient after patient with very similar profiles, I realized that simple education could touch many lives. I joined a small group of committed individuals who collectively worked with the South Texas Chapter of the American Heart Association (AHA), and we laid the groundwork for an annual educational luncheon on the topic of heart disease in women; the luncheon was open to the public, and many of my patients attended. This was in 1996, way before Diet Coke cans started carrying the swishy "Go Red" logo and heart disease, the number one killer of women, got any play in the media. Heart disease just lurked as a silent threat, and I worked tirelessly to bring the disease the focus it deserved. I went out into the Texas community to churches, women's groups, and public forums to educate and empower women with ideas—everything from hosting healthy cooking parties to setting up neighborhood walking groups—to foster a healthier lifestyle.

Our family, including three kids under the age of five, then headed to Halifax, Nova Scotia, in 1998, where my husband had a two-year fellowship. Again, I found extreme cardiac cases; in Nova Scotia, like the rest of Canada, 31 percent of all deaths are due to heart disease, and every seven minutes somebody dies from heart disease or a stroke, according to the Heart and Stroke Foundation of Nova Scotia. The women I saw were referred to me by their primary care doctors and had basically given up on their health. They felt that their family history of heart disease was a death sentence and they couldn't do anything about it. So they made unhealthy choices like smoking, consuming foods high in saturated fats, and not making an effort to exercise. Depression was also prevalent among these patients, and I knew firsthand that getting these people motivated to exercise was about as close to a magic bullet as I would ever have. I organized a three-mile Mother-Daughter Walk for Heart Disease that raised awareness about the disease in Nova Scotia. As I stood on the podium with Caitlin, my then three-year-old daughter, and addressed the crowd before the walk, I realized that working to help women improve their lives and their health was going to be an important part of my life, wherever I happened to be living and working.

During my time in Nova Scotia, I was frequently invited to speak to women's groups about heart health. Through my public speaking to women's groups, I got the community of women moving and directed them to resources already existing within their communities that would help them tackle their inactivity and poor nutrition as well as the stressful situations many of them lived in day to day.

While in Nova Scotia, I had the opportunity to reach out to aboriginal Canadians (a group known to be commonly affected by diabetes, high blood pressure, obesity, and heart disease) through a series of educational seminars at a tribal meeting. Dressed in a suit and heels, I walked into the smoke-filled room (the smoking ban was nonexistent then) and felt totally out of place. At first, the crowd, most of whom were wearing faded jeans and sweatshirts, didn't listen; they assumed they would have no connection to me. Then I shared my history with them: my maternal grandmother was born on a reservation in Oklahoma to a Pawnee Indian mother and white father. She spent her early life in poverty but grew to be a nurturing woman who was one of the major influences on my life. Once I had the group's attention, I shared with them the knowledge that there were resources in Halifax that could help with the burden of health and social problems that plagued their community, which included diabetes, alcoholism, depression, and heart disease. Historically, this aboriginal community was untrusting of the traditional medical system and was prone to neglect, if not outright ignore, their health problems.

My message to the crowd that day was that they, in fact, had control over their lives—which was easy to say but harder for them to do. I told them that to take the reins, they had to make a few tough choices like tossing out the cigarettes and choosing a walk over a six-pack of beer. I received a highly emotional and powerful letter after my presentation, relating the overwhelmingly positive response of the audience to my comments. Two years in Nova Scotia wasn't long enough to truly become entrenched with those lovely people, but I certainly hope that a few lives were changed for the better.

My deep South and true North experiences allowed me to find my calling as a doctor: through communication, or more specifically, by listening and relating to people, I could transform lives. Although my training had prepared me to spend my time doing surgical heart procedures like injecting dye to look at heart arteries and opening blocked arteries with stents, I realized that I would have a much better chance at changing my patients' lives by focusing on preventing disease before it happened. I shifted my focus from interventional cardiology, where most of my time was spent in the laboratory, to noninvasive cardiology, including patient care, reading heart ultrasounds, and doing research.

Back to 2006: My cancer turned out to be treatable, so now it was time to take care of the rest of my life. Taking Kelly's message to heart, I started living the way I had always wanted to—meaning I wouldn't sweat the small stuff anymore, I'd build a life that was consistent with my priorities, and I would live actively, not passively. Not everything was perfect (as if it ever is for anyone!), but I analyzed my priorities and targeted which areas needed work. I had to learn how to set limits, say no, and spend my time and effort working toward things that were important to me and to my family. I found my voice and learned that my skills of effective communication, honed during public-speaking classes in high school, could allow me to educate other women and their care providers on a much larger scale. I sought to rid myself of the anxiety that had plagued me since separating from my husband. When I became newly single, worry was my closest friend. I worried about money, my kids, my parents, my job, and balancing all of my personal and professional commitments. I met with a mental health counselor and learned to face my fears directly and create solutions to the problems in front of me.

I traveled to Tibet in the fall of 2006, just before my diagnosis, and observed how happy and peaceful the nomads were despite the fact that each person carried everything that they owned in one small bag. I tried to incorporate their spirit of family, generosity, and belief in a higher power to help me out of my rut. I reached out to the love and friendship around me by reconnecting with friends from my past and appreciating the friends and loved ones who were part of my daily life. I basked in the knowledge that I did have the power to make things better in my life. I started practicing yoga regularly, streamlined my diet, and spent time outdoors with my children hiking, swimming, and kayaking. Within months I really started to feel better inside and out. I was beginning to recover from the sad events that had touched my life and was ready to take on challenges to nurture my soul.

I had already planted the seeds of the HAPPY Heart study earlier that year, and firmly believed it would create great things. Ironically, I spent the weekend after learning I had breast cancer writing a grant to obtain funding for the project. When I originally conceived of the idea, funding for this kind of project on the scale that we would need to start was nearly impossible to find. A friend once told me, "After you commit, the Universe conspires to make things happen." Happen they did. I received word that a benefactor had come forth who wanted to make a large grant to fund this project in memory of a loved one who had died in her fifties from undiagnosed heart disease. Talk about turning tragedy into triumph: the money donated by this family has touched hundreds of lives already by allowing almost seventy women to enroll in the program. Each of these women has a child, spouse, sibling, parent, or friend who also benefits from the improved health and happiness gained from participating in the trial.

The generosity of the Universe didn't stop there. Through a contact at my hospital, I was introduced to the director of the community health center in Revere, Massachusetts, which coincidentally was opening the first wellness center for low-income families in our network. This center was to become the home to HAPPY Heart. A unique group of inspiring and passionate nurses, nutritionists, and physical therapists—professionals who knew the community and the challenges faced by its residents—quickly agreed to work with the study. Together we designed an innovative study that would do what no research had done before: take a group of women with enormous health challenges in their lives and through a variety of methods—group education, support from a peer group, a team of health coaches, and participation in mind-body therapies—improve both their emotional and physical health and, in doing so, significantly reduce their risk for cardiovascular disease.

I sat among a group of low-income, stress-laden, weary women at our first HAPPY Heart meeting and definitely looked out of place. I am sure they thought we had little in common, just as the Latinas in Texas and the Aborigines in Canada had. But as I related the challenges I had faced, both in 2006 and beyond, the women started to realize that we were more alike than different. I shared my philosophy both as a survivor and as a physician: we all face challenges large and small, but there is no challenge we cannot handle with a supportive network of friends and family, and the right attitude.

I explained to the women in the study that while we cannot change many of the circumstances in our lives, we can create a life that brings us emotional clarity and improved health. We worked with the women to help them recognize that they deserved time to focus on themselves—no cell phones, spouses, or children—during which they could concentrate on healing their hearts and dipping their toes into the pool of peace and tranquility. We reminded them that the house wouldn't fall down if they took a few extra hours a week to attend a tai chi class, laughter yoga, or educational session. The women slowly started warming up to their health coaches and peers and began implementing the health, behavior, and lifestyle strategies that we share in this book. Ever so gradually, the pounds started to come off, the attitudes improved, and smiles crept onto everyone's faces. The women still have obstacles, of course, but now they laugh and live life with joy . . . as, thankfully, do I.

chapter one

Smart at Heart

It's a Monday night, a few weeks before Christmas. Around 5:30, thirteen women file into a conference room at the Massachusetts General Hospital (MGH) Revere Health Center in Revere, Massachusetts. Some grab a clementine from a table of healthy snacks, while others peel off the layers they'd been wearing to protect themselves from the bitter wind coming off the Atlantic Ocean one hundred yards away. Of the thirteen, nine are participants in HAPPY Heart, a two-year-old program that integrates all the facets of a woman's life (including, among other things, physical health, emotional well-being, stress levels, and relationships) to minimize her cardiac-related issues. Three of the women are nurses (or *health coaches*, in HAPPY-Heart speak) and one is a daughter of a participant. As the group begins to settle into seats around the table, Isabel, one HAPPY Hearter, announces that she's going to gather clothes for the homeless in the next week and pass them out and is looking for donations of any size. Another participant, Jenny, mentions that her daughter is taking finals, and that those tests have the whole house stressed out. A third subject, Kim, has an ankle that's hurting, and Donna Peltier-Saxe, one of the health coaches, promises to take a look at it later.

Donna Slicis, another health coach, sets up her computer, and the first PowerPoint slide shows on a screen. "Family: The Good, The Bad, and The Ugly," it reads, "Holiday survival!" After a few introductory remarks, Slicis, who has a great sense of humor and an even bigger sense of compassion, shows a YouTube video, which is called "Family Survival Kit." The infomercial parody "sells" such helpful items as criticism-canceling headphones and Dr. Phil in a can. ("You can't change what you don't acknowledge," the bald doc preaches from within the aluminum walls.) Laughter and nods of, "So true, so true" fill the room. The mood is light as Slicis focuses on the bulk of her presentation: creating a holiday experience that is low on conflict and bad health habits, and high on self-care.

Self-care is a relatively new topic for the women here tonight. "I've never taken care of my health," says Lucy, echoing the sentiments of many in the group. "I just hoped for the best." Revere is a blue-collar town, and for most of these women's lives, the natural order of basic human needs—food and water, a safe place to live and sleep, a steady income—dictated that their energy and effort be put toward simply surviving as opposed to thriving. One woman is dealing with a foreclosure on her house; another, at age forty-nine, has had to move back in with her mother because she lost her job and can't afford her own place. One was shot by a former boyfriend and still has three bullets in her body, while another woman has a son who is a heroin addict. Understandably, self-care hasn't been a priority for these women; they've been too busy figuring out how to pay the bills, put food on their tables, deal with abusive relationships, and just generally navigate the messy details of life. "My life has never been about me," says Heather, mother of the addicted son. "I've spent it taking care of my mother, my siblings, my children, my husband. I never thought to put myself first."

Those life circumstances, combined with their family health histories, put most of them at risk for cardiovascular disease. To be a participant in the HAPPY Heart study, candidates have to have at least two major risk factors for cardiovascular disease: high blood pressure, abnormal cholesterol levels, diabetes, obesity, cigarette smoking, sedentary lifestyle, and genetic history of cardiac issues in the family. Over 80 percent of the sixty-five women in the program have at least three risk factors; the most common are obesity, low levels of HDL (the good kind of cholesterol), and a sedentary lifestyle.

Unfortunately, the women are in good company. The American Heart Association (AHA) issued new guidelines for the prevention of cardiovascular disease in women in early 2011, and the statistics cited in the introduction are troubling—to say the least. Two in three women over the age of thirty are either overweight or obese. More than twelve million American women have diabetes, a disease that is so tightly linked to cardiovascular disease that doctors often treat the two conditions simultaneously. Many physicians now refer to diabetes and obesity as "diabesity," because of their frequent coexistence. High blood pressure is on the rise, especially among African-American women; an overwhelming 44 percent of that population has high blood pressure.

Although two of the most popular American pastimes—eating fast food and spending extended periods of time in front of a screen—might lead you to think otherwise, the epidemic of cardiovascular disease is not limited to the United States. "Heart disease is the leading cause of death in women in every major developed country and most emerging economies," the 2011 AHA report proclaims.[1]

Given that heart disease is the number one killer of women—in the United States in 2006, over 430,000 women died from cardiovascular disease while about 270,000 died from various forms of cancer—the public awareness is still disturbingly low.[2] In the AHA guidelines, researchers found that only 53 percent of women polled said that the first thing they would do if they suspected they were having a heart attack would be to call 911.[3] That lack of awareness, combined with the rise of obesity, is contributing to a trend that shouldn't be happening in the twenty-first century: death rates from cardiovascular disease for women under the age of fifty-four are, amazingly, rising. For the first time in forty years, the number of U.S. women between ages thirty-five and fifty-four who die from heart-related issues is actually increasing.[4]

As is true for many women across the world, the threat of a cardiac event stares down the HAPPY Heart participants daily. "My father died of arterial sclerosis at sixty-two," says Christie, sixty years old, one of the participants who heard about the program from me when she came to my office with heart palpitations. "And my mother was a diabetic who had a triple bypass and a pacemaker. Seven of her siblings died of heart problems before [heart disease] took her at age eighty. Those thoughts just live in the back of my head."

Daily challenges don't loom so large tonight, though. Tonight, these women—like most of America—are preparing for two weeks of holiday excess: large, rich meals; champagne, eggnog, and plenty of other drinks; intense family time; additional cooking and cleaning; and unspoken, and often huge, expectations. The situation is a recipe for total meltdown for anybody, so Slicis encourages people to forget about perfection. "Be realistic about your expectations," she says. "If the potatoes don't come out perfectly, nobody will notice but you." Then she moves on to talk about more important matters, which include how to protect yourself and your feelings around a group of people who might not always be the most supportive and loving. "You get to be happy even if everybody else around you isn't," she says, adding that it's important to walk away from negative conversations and take a time-out if need be. "The bathroom is a great place to hide," she says with a laugh. After touching on some budget-minded gifts (a family cookbook, certificates for closet organizing), Slicis reminds everyone to go for walks, get enough sleep, and to remember that a holiday is one day. "It's not a holi-week or a holi-month, so celebrate accordingly," she says. The group laughs in agreement.

The holiday survival tips, the hummus and other healthy snacks, and the women who are here tonight are all part of a common goal: building a heart that is strong and healthy in every respect. Although it may seem like cardiovascular disease is best treated by doctors in white coats, medical care is just one piece of the puzzle. Sure, doctors can monitor your cholesterol and your glucose levels, your weight and your blood pressure, but your cardiovascular—and overall—health depends on so much more than simple measurements.

I firmly believe—and science has proven—that getting smart at heart is about evaluating your whole life, from your relationships to your environment to your mental state. "Medications alone aren't enough. Surgical procedures aren't enough. Stents aren't enough," says Kate Traynor, a colleague of mine and the program director at the Cardiovascular Disease Prevention Center at MGH in Boston. "How many times have you heard that somebody needs to go back for another stent? Where the rubber hits the road—and what will keep you and your heart healthy—are lifestyle changes."

In addition to the more obvious factors like diet and exercise, research shows that your cardiac health is influenced, among other things, by how much stress is in your life, and more importantly, how you deal with it; the strength of your friendships and family connections (or the lack of them); the quality of the sleep you do or don't get; your perspective on the world. In other words, defusing toxic relationships is as important to your heart as easing up on the butter in the mashed potatoes. And getting your house in order to receive guests is as key to good health as taking daily walks.

When I care for a patient, I don't treat a number, a heart, or a disease; I treat a person. Similarly, when I put together the premise for HAPPY Heart, I wanted to address individuals and all the aspects of their complicated, challenging lives—not just the ones that usually get discussed in my cardiology office. I can only see a handful of patients daily, though, and the HAPPY Heart ladies are in the greater Boston area; I wanted to share my message with as many people as possible, which is how this book came to be.

A Quick Course in Human Physiology

Before we discuss heart health any further, I want you to have a basic idea of how the heart functions, as well as how the rest of your body reacts to everyday emotions and life. I am a big believer that knowledge is power, and many of the patients I see have not taken ownership of their health, which means they'll never feel empowered enough to believe they can make meaningful, effective changes. "Some women take more time and better care of their fingernails than they do of their heart," says Slicis with a laugh. "They spent ten minutes picking out a polish color and can tell you the whole process of acrylics, but they don't understand what their cholesterol levels mean."

The heart, which is technically a muscle, starts to beat not long after conception and continues working until the very last breath somebody takes; over the course of an average lifetime, it will beat over 2.5 billion times. The heart consists of four chambers: two *atria*, which receive blood, and two *ventricles*, which pump blood. Between the chambers are *valves*, which serve as doors, opening and closing to keep the blood moving forward. *Blue blood*, or oxygen-depleted blood, flows from the body to the right atrium, through the tricuspid valve, and into the right ventricle. Exiting through the pulmonary artery, it heads to the lungs to lose the carbon dioxide it's carrying and to become oxygenated and red. It returns to the left atrium, through the left ventricle, and on to the aorta, which sends it out into the body. The *aorta* is the tree trunk of the body; many arteries, arterioles, and capillaries branch off it, getting progressively smaller in size so that blood can be delivered to all the organs and tissues in the body. The blood then returns to the heart via *venules* that lead into veins.

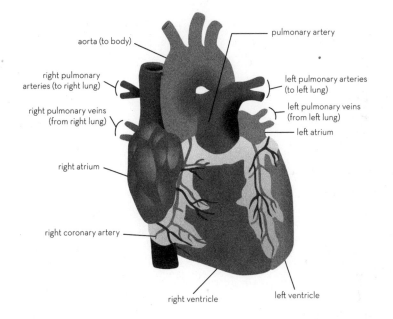

aorta (to body)

pulmonary artery

right pulmonary arteries (to right lung)

left pulmonary arteries (to left lung)

right pulmonary veins (from right lung)

left pulmonary veins (from left lung)

left atrium

right atrium

right coronary artery

right ventricle

left ventricle

The pumping of a heart is an incredibly intricate process. By using new detailed imaging techniques, doctors have learned that it doesn't just squeeze with every beat—it also twists and untwists. Those motions, in combination with electrical signals and blood pressure, combine to form a rhythm that cycles blood through your heart seventy times a minute while you're at rest and sends roughly one hundred gallons of blood every hour through your body.

We are born with arteries that are clean and clear, but over time we intentionally and unintentionally expose ourselves to substances that encourage the formation of blockages or plaques within the arteries (or as my grandmother used to call it, "hardening of the arteries"). *Plaques* are composed of lipids, fat, and scar tissue. A few factors known to initiate and worsen plaque development include high cholesterol, smoking, diabetes, and high blood pressure. In many cases the plaque lining the arteries is filled with a soft fatty core, which makes the plaque highly susceptible to rupturing. When that happens, that inner core attracts blood platelets and blood cells and a clot appears, which results in partial or complete blockage of the artery, which in turn leads to a heart attack. In some people—and in women in particular—the plaque doesn't rupture entirely but instead erodes or is scraped open. In these situations, platelets still accumulate, but the buildup doesn't necessarily obstruct the blood flow through the artery. It does, however, decrease the flow enough to cause some degree of heart muscle damage and symptoms of chest discomfort.

The organ with the four chambers that I just described? That's your physical heart. As you might guess, it's not the only heart I consider when I examine a patient. Harder to quantify but just as integral to good health is what I call the *emotional heart*. This side of the heart gets brought up regularly in everyday conversations, through common phrases like *you have a big heart; let's get to the heart of the matter; she is the heart and soul of this business; that was heart wrenching; he has hardened his heart.* Translating that language, it's clear we believe that the heart signifies a place where spirit lives, where purpose is found, where emotion begins and settles. The love, disappointment, contentment, fear, and euphoria we feel deeply within our hearts seems to ricochet through the body; while watching a frightening movie or hearing unbelievably good news, your heart seems to beat so rapidly, it almost echoes in your ears.

While the physical heart is the team captain for the circulatory system, the emotional heart is more of a team player—its health is influenced by other parts of the body, and vice versa. An important teammate to the emotional heart is the brain. Your brain responds to emotions by activating systems in your body that release various compounds and create a change in how your body is functioning.

For instance, when you're watching that scary movie, your body shifts into the *fight-or-flight response*, a natural reaction that happens when you feel threatened. In fight or flight, the brain signals the adrenal glands to send out adrenaline, noradrenaline, dopamine, and cortisol that cause your heart to beat faster and your blood pressure and blood glucose levels to rise. These phenomena put your body into an aggressive, ultraprepared mode, even though the biggest threat you're really facing is choking on your popcorn. There doesn't have to be a monster haunting your thoughts for your body to react unfavorably to emotions. The trigger can be a parent who is entering a bad spell of health, a boss who requires working on the weekend, or anybody or anything that brings stress into your life.

Fortunately, the brain also controls the release of chemicals that can have positive effects on our health and mood. *Neurotransmitters* are chemical messengers that allow nerve cells to communicate with one another. Here are four important ones:

- *Serotonin* positively influences how we feel, learn, think, and sleep.

- *Dopamine*, at lower doses than those released in the fight-or-flight response, provides feelings of enjoyment and is central to motivation and movement.

- *Endorphins* are the euphoria-producing neurotransmitters mainly responsible for the so-called runner's high after exercise. (They're also released during orgasm.)

- *Oxytocin*, commonly known as the "love hormone," is released during sexual attraction, orgasm, and when people see pictures of those with whom they are in love. It also provides contented, relaxed, and trusting feelings.

That overview just touches on the basics of the two hearts; I'll delve into them more deeply in chapter 2, devoted to physical health, and chapter 3, which covers emotional health. For now, the most important thing to remember is that everything about your health is interrelated; just as I can't fully treat high blood pressure without looking at a person's lifestyle and circumstances, one system in the body also affects the other ones.

Connecting the Physical
and Emotional Hearts

One of my patients, Mary, a hard-working paraprofessional in the financial world, was in her early sixties and looking forward to retirement with her husband of over thirty years. Before either of them could cash in a 401(k) though, he had a heart attack while gardening and died within a few hours. Within twelve hours of her beloved passing away, Mary, who was thirty pounds overweight, with borderline diabetes and high blood pressure, was admitted to the hospital with what seemed like a heart attack.

Fortunately, it was not. Instead, a surge of adrenaline, brought on by the trauma of losing her husband, caused the bottom half of her heart muscle to blow up like a balloon and temporarily stop functioning, which then forced the top half of her heart to pick up the slack and work twice as hard. Medically, the condition is called *apical ballooning*, but it's more commonly known as broken heart syndrome: when your grief is so great, your heart mimics the symptoms of a heart attack.

Affecting a small part of the population—and mostly postmenopausal women—a broken heart is part of our lexicon.[5] We say you can die of a broken heart—and, as Mary almost proved, that can be true. Broken heart syndrome is just one example of the strong correlation between the emotional and physical hearts. That said, you don't have to lose a loved one to have a heart that is injured by your emotions. Unemployment, financial uncertainty, an unsupportive spouse, a lack of focus and purpose, unmitigated stress, and a host of other situations can send a heart on an unhealthy path, as recent studies have proven:

- The ups and downs of the recession have shown a marked influence on the number of cases of heart attacks. Studying the data from the Duke University Databank for Cardiovascular Disease in conjunction with the U.S. stock market performance, researchers in 2010 found a significant increase in heart attack rates during a seven-month period of stock market decrease.[6]

- The correlation isn't just an American phenomenon either. Studying the same relationship for two years and publishing results in 2010, Chinese doctors found similar results with the Shanghai Stock Exchange Composite Index. "Both the rising and falling of the Index were associated with more deaths, and the fewest deaths coincided with little or no change of the Index," they concluded, noting that a 100-point change in the Index corresponded to a 5.17 percent increase in coronary heart disease deaths.[7]

- Research stemming from the INTERHEART Study, a globally based study that includes over twenty-seven thousand participants in fifty-two countries, is scientifically proving what we long thought to be true: stress and depression, combined with other established risk factors, can increase one's risk of heart attack significantly. One study, based solely on Chinese participants, found that depression and permanent stress put people at risk for a heart attack, while a broader study that reflected international data documented nine modifiable risk factors, which included everything from diabetes to smoking.[8] The results were invaluable; for the first time in 2008, stress was included in a very solid, comprehensive study.

- Looking at eighteen women who had either lost a mother or sister to breast cancer within five years, researchers in 2009 measured the relationship between proteins known to be associated with inflammation (cytokines) released by cells that are associated with infection, disease, low mood and motivation, and brain activation in the areas responsible for emotional processing. They were the first researchers to find a marked relationship between those two components: strong activity in the emotional part of the brain increased the levels of harmful cytokines.[9]

- In another study, released in 2011, a team of psychologists recruited forty people who had experienced an unwanted romantic breakup within the previous six months; the breakups were not initiated by these participants. During one part of the study, they were asked to look at a picture of their ex and think about how they felt by being rejected; during another, they were given a minor irritation on their forearm, akin to holding a hot cup of coffee. The researchers took functional *magnetic resonance imaging* (MRI) scans of their brains during both tasks and found that both activated the regions of the brain that are involved in physical pain.[10] This study illustrates the important link between our emotions, our brain, and our perception of physical pain, and explains why many of us experience physical pain in the setting of significant rejection.

I see these negative emotional-physical heart connections frequently in both my patients and HAPPY Heart participants. For example, my patient Anna had a bullying male boss, which caused her severe anxiety and destroyed her self-confidence. Over the course of a year, she gained thirty pounds, had to take increasingly higher doses of medications to control her blood pressure, and developed severe insomnia. Eventually, on the brink of a breakdown, she filed a complaint and got switched to another department. Within months, she shed all her new pounds, her blood pressure returned to normal, and so did her sleeping habits. Her belligerent boss had caused her body to remain constantly in the fight-or-flight mode, which changed the way it completed basic functions like metabolizing food and sleeping. In other words, she lost her health because of him.

As Anna proves, the information highway between your emotional and physical hearts travels both ways. Your emotions can make you sick, but they can also enhance your well-being. The proof of this has been a hot topic in science lately:

- Just as scary movies can send your body into fight-or-flight syndrome, comedies—and the accompanying joyous laughter— can relax your cardiovascular system. In 2010, a group of researchers had seventeen adults watch either a comedy or documentary for thirty minutes on separate days. When they were watching the comedy, their heart rates and blood pressure increased, and the blood vessels opened up, increasing blood flow (a good thing; they tightened up during the documentary).

- Additionally, a different marker of a healthy blood vessel response, the softness of the carotid artery—another good thing—increased after watching the comedy and didn't return to its baseline reading until twenty-four hours after watching—whereas it did not change significantly throughout viewing of the documentary. In other words, to repeat a cliché, laughter is the best kind of medicine. This study demonstrates that not only do our brains feel better in the presence of a good laugh, so do our hearts.[11]

- Andrew Steptoe, PhD, a psychology professor at the University of London, is a pioneer in the field of emotion and physical wellness. Through his multiple studies that involve ten thousand middle-aged men and women, he has repeatedly concluded that the happier a person is, the less *cortisol* (a stress-related hormone; more on that in chapter 4) they produce; the lower their blood pressure and heart rate are; and the fewer the markers of inflammation, which is tied to diseases like cancer, heart disease, asthma, arthritis, and other autoimmune disorders.[12] Looking at the risk of death as a single entity, Steptoe and some colleagues performed a review of studies evaluating a sense of positive well-being (which included descriptions like *joy, happiness, vigor, energy, hopefulness, sense of humor,* and *life satisfaction*) and risk of death. In both healthy and unhealthy individuals, they found that a sense of optimism is associated with a decreased risk of dying.[13]

- In 2010, researchers at Brigham Young University and the University of North Carolina at Chapel Hill conducted a comprehensive analysis of health and relationships. Compiling data from 148 studies that involved more than three hundred thousand people worldwide, the team found that people with weak social connections had on average 50 percent higher odds of death in the study's follow-up period (an average of seven-and-a-half years) than people with more solid connections. That improvement in lifespan is equal to the impact of quitting smoking.[14]

- Researchers at Case Western Reserve University pulled together all the studies they could find that looked at altruism, or helping others, and the effect on well-being, health, and longevity. Among other benefits they document, they refer to the "helper's high," a positive physical sensation that occurs as a result of volunteering or aiding others; other emotions that were associated with helping include feeling stronger, more energetic, warm, calmer, and less depressed, greater self-worth, and fewer aches and pains. They also talk about the possibility that positive emotions essentially shove out negative ones. "It is difficult to be angry, resentful, or fearful when one is showing unselfish love toward another person," they write. Although they mention the need for further research, they conclude that "A generous life is a happier and healthier one."[15]

Happiness Defined

Although my study is called HAPPY Heart, happiness isn't exactly what I am—or you should—be after in your quest for better health. The word *happy* has a connotation that implies that a person is always smiling, unfazed by the troubles that life throws at them. Obviously, that's far from realistic for anybody.

More accurate than *happiness* are words like *well-being, satisfaction*, or *contentment*. In fact, one of the questions researchers used to gauge happiness in the happiness–blood pressure study was, "Would you say you are very satisfied, fairly satisfied, not very satisfied, or not at all satisfied with the life you lead?" Satisfaction or a positive outlook connotes a much more universal, enduring perspective, not just random moments of bliss or enjoyment. While the ups and downs of daily life—everything from the frustration you feel when you can't find your keys to the elation you feel when you are given a raise—might give you small emotional bumps one way or the other, your perceived quality of life isn't based on the events of one day. Instead, it is based on a decades-long view of your life experience and relationships.

Implicit in the idea of being content or satisfied is the belief that a content person generally has a positive perspective on life. What makes you able to see a glass—or your life—half full instead of half empty? Despite what many may think, it's not wealth, prestige, or power. In their classic book, *Character Strengths and Virtues: A Handbook and Classification*, psychologists Christopher Peterson and Martin Seligman list the personal traits that seem to be most closely associated with a positive outlook on life. They include persistence, creativity, kindness, prudence, humility, leadership, and the ability to love and learn. Appreciation of beauty and striving for excellence were other positive traits they recognized as beneficial for creating and maintaining a sense of contentment.[16] Using those criteria, the women in HAPPY Heart, despite having tough lives on paper, have immensely positive outlooks. They have great persistence, battling uphill against their health, and all exhibit humility and kindness, among other traits, in their own unique ways.

The HAPPY Heart program helped many of the women change their outlooks. "I came into this group thinking life is just happening to me and I have no control," says Joyce, one of the participants who has basically done a 180-degree turn with her life. "This group has totally altered my perception of myself, and my life." Joyce isn't an exception to an unbreakable rule that says your life satisfaction is out of your hands. Like most everything else I will talk about in this book, it most definitely is in your control.

Science has proven this. While moods can change from day to day—and from one minute to the next—psychologists used to believe that life satisfaction remained stable over time, always returning to a set point after a traumatic or joyous event. A 2005 study, published in the *Journal of Personality and Social Psychology*, challenged that notion. Two psychologists analyzed various data from over 3,600 participants over seventeen years, and found that nearly one in four people's rating of their *life satisfaction* (LS) changed significantly from the first five years of the study to the last five years. In fact, life satisfaction ratings were shifted so regularly, the authors write, "Height, weight, body mass index, . . . blood pressure, and personality traits were all more stable than LS."[17]

Translation: Even if you are known as a negative person or if you can't seem to cultivate strong friendships or if you feel like you continually pick the wrong partner for a relationship, that doesn't necessarily mean that's the way it's always going to be. In fact, you've picked up the perfect book to help you switch things up.

Your Toolbox

Believing so deeply in the power within each of us to live a happier, healthier life, I wanted to provide as many tools as possible for the sixty-five women in the HAPPY Heart program to connect their physical and emotional hearts. When they enroll in the program, each woman gets a consultation with a physical therapist, a registered dietician, and a health coach who helps each set attainable, smart goals for herself. Their stats—blood pressure, weight, height, cholesterol, waist circumference—are measured and monitored regularly. In addition, the women have access to free exercise programs like yoga and tai chi and reduced-fee alternative therapies such as acupuncture and massage. Finally, the Monday night meetings, which cover everything from excessive belly fat to public speaking, are a venue for education, as well as confidence and friendship building. Basically, I think of HAPPY Heart as a boot camp for these women's lives.

The success of a holistic, group approach to healing has been documented in a similar study held at Ohio State University. In that study, researchers followed 227 women who were surgically treated for breast cancer. Half of them were put into small groups that received weekly instructional sessions devoted to topics like reducing stress, improving mood, changing health behavior, and adhering to cancer treatment and care. The other half was simply left to their own devices. After four months, the patients who had the weekly sessions had less anxiety and better nutritional habits, smoked less, and felt more socially supported than the group who didn't receive support. Their physical symptoms improved as well; the women in the intervention group demonstrated enhanced immune function, which paralleled their psychological and behavioral improvements.[18] This study emphasizes the importance of receiving important health education information in the setting of a supportive group. The group dynamic and support increased the ability of the participants to make positive health choices.

Initially, we were going to set up HAPPY Heart in a similar way: as a controlled study, with half of the women receiving the health coaching and support while the other half would simply have their blood and physiological markers measured. After we discussed the implications at length, I didn't have the heart not to give every participant a comprehensive approach to cardiovascular care. I could guess what the outcome of the study would be, and I didn't like the idea of setting up half of the women to most likely fail. Instead, we restructured the study so that each woman's improvement could be compared to her baseline state. That way we could give everybody equal access to support—and success.

While this book can't physically transport you to Revere for boot camp, it can virtually transport you there. Working with the women in HAPPY Heart and the many women I have cared for over the past two decades has given me the insight to see what works and what doesn't in the process of empowering women to make sometimes difficult—but potentially lifesaving—changes in their lives. This book not only will provide the necessary information and ideas about steps you need to take but will also help you better understand how to make these changes in your own busy life. I have dug up all the current research and combined it with my experience; in doing so, I've created a comprehensive, hands-on book that gives you access to the many (power) tools I have in my arsenal, ranging from nutritional tips from HAPPY Heart health coaches to detailed information about surprising causes of high blood pressure.

The combination of translated medical information and easy-to-access advice has helped the HAPPY Heart women thrive. Over two years, we've seen steady improvements that range from weight loss (one patient lost 10" from her waist, 8" from her hips, and 1.5" from her neck; we measure inches as well as pounds because abdominal fat is such a huge factor in cardiovascular disease) to attitudes ("Every day feels like Christmas to me now. Seriously," says one participant who, I'm pretty sure, smiles even when she's sleeping). "I now think to myself, 'What are you doing to improve yourself?'" says

Joyce, reflecting on her new perspective: "Am I taking time to care for myself? Have I taken a deep breath today? Have I exercised? Have I put myself first at all this whole week?"

This book will teach you how to care for yourself, and your heart; how to take deep breaths, and why you need them; how to make exercise something you enjoy, not dread; and how to put yourself first this week, and the next week, and the next.

To become smart at heart, you have to address ten major components that bridge the gap between your physical heart and your emotional heart. I visualize it this way: Your physical heart is on one side of an imaginary river and your emotional heart is on the other, and there are ten bridges that connect the two.

Here are the ten bridges that connect the two hearts:

- **Physical health:** the state of your four-chambered heart as well as the rest of your body

- **Emotional health:** the condition of your emotional heart, your feelings, how you process them, and the influence they have on your health

- **Stress management:** how you handle the push and pull of daily life and how that affects your body

- **Exercise:** the importance of moving your body regularly and with purpose

- **Nutrition:** the significance of diet, and consuming healthy foods in a mindful way

- **Relationships:** the connections with your immediate family, close friends, and others in your inner circle

- **Communication:** the myriad ways you send messages to the world, including talking, body language, and self-talk
- **Environment:** the "health" of the places you spend most of your time: your home, your workplace, your car
- **Mindfulness:** the importance of quiet, quality time to enhance your health
- **Modification:** ways to effectively make the changes we've suggested in this book

I have devoted one chapter to each bridge. The first two chapters, the physical health and emotional health bridges, are mostly informational, as I feel you need a basic understanding of the way the body and mind work to be able to cross the other eight bridges effectively.

Does this list feel overwhelming? Don't let it, even if you feel like you've hit a dead end with your health. I will never forget a handful of patients I have encountered who had basically given up and accepted a death sentence. They had looks of resignation upon their faces and a lack of hope in the tone of their voices. They were ready to give in, having made the conscious decision to just go along for the ride as opposed to being an active participant in their own lives.

I shared with these patients that just as Dorothy always had the power to get back to Kansas within her, they also have the power within themselves to change their lives. It simply involves making the conscious decision to pull their heads out of the sand, to face the adversities at hand, and to recognize and embrace all the good in their lives. By taking the proper steps, they could go from being hopeless to hopeful, and improved health would likely follow.

Before We Get Started

Before we go about making you smart at heart, there are two important things I emphasize with my patients and in the HAPPY Heart program. I want you to know them too:

1. The first is that you are the most important health care provider on your team. "Women need to feel empowered to be the day-to-day decision maker[s] when it comes to their health," says Susan Lane, RN, MSN, MBA, a health educator in HAPPY Heart. "You are in charge of your health on a daily basis, not just when you're feeling bad or in a doctor's office." Certainly a doctor and her advice can be an instrumental part of your decision-making process, but only you know how you feel and only you can make yourself feel better. Put in a simpler way, "You can drive the bus," says Donna Saxe-Peltier, using one of her favorite empowering phrases.

2. The second thing is that all advice comes without judgment of your past. We've all made mistakes, health-related or otherwise, and there's no reason to dwell on them. "Here is who you are today," says Susan Lane, explaining the philosophy we use. "Let's make who you are today feel better."

I don't expect a life overhaul in thirty days—and I'm not promising that either. I'm not going to force you to quit smoking or give up cupcakes or start running. "You come in whatever window or door you can get in," says Susan, and I love that idea: we meet you where you are. I have four kids, basically work two jobs, and have plenty of other obligations. Between managing my family and my career, I realize how complicated and busy life can very quickly get. I also realize that your daily routines, from your choice of breakfast food to where you dump your purse when you get home, are firmly engrained.

But I am going to give you the scientific evidence on why it is important to cut out cigarettes, eat right, move your body, and make other life changes that will be hugely beneficial. Then I'll gently suggest ways to get on a healthy path that connects your physical and emotional hearts. The strategies I offer have been successful for all of my patients, whether they're HAPPY Heart ones or people I see through my regular clinical practice. They're based on my belief that small steps and changes can echo through your body with surprising speed, creating a whole heart and a healthier you.

Yes, it will take some work, but you picked up this book for a reason. You know it's time to make some changes, to (finally) put yourself and your health on your to-do list, to improve your life in small, but very important and tangible ways. In other words, it's time to get smart at heart.

chapter two

The Physical Health Bridge

As a cardiologist who spends most of my days with a stethoscope around my neck, the physical heart—and all the systems that support it—are never far from my mind.

In many ways, the physical health bridge is the easiest bridge of the ten bridges to address: I can count a patient's heartbeats and look at her numbers for blood pressure and feel her pulse. Unlike a person's relationships, stress level, or communication style, physical health is pretty black-and-white; I can read a patient's chart, without her being in front of me, and know what kind of health she is in. Looking for participants in the HAPPY Heart program, we used heart disease risk factors to get our group; having two or more risk factors was the price of admission. Even though we knew that we were going to address all aspects of their lives, physical traits are the most concrete way to measure somebody's health.

In many other ways, identifying areas that need work in the physical bridge and putting them in proper order is a substantial challenge. Chances are, you have spent your life reinforcing habits that you are now going to change. This takes time, motivation, and, most importantly, patience. Changes in blood pressure, cholesterol, and weight don't come overnight. I won't lie: you have your work cut out for you. The good news, however, is that you will reap the rewards of these changes for the rest of your life.

Your physical health is obviously a major bridge when it comes to cardiovascular health. If it breaks, this bridge can be one of the hardest to repair. Being smart at heart starts with assessing the body in which you live, and I have devoted much of this chapter to helping you understand everything from cholesterol to C-reactive proteins. This knowledge will help you as you cross the bridges in chapters 3 to 11.

Warning Signs of Heart Disease, Heart Attack, and Stroke Response

When most people think of a heart attack, they think of the movie version: a man develops sudden onset of a feeling of a weight on his chest and falls to the floor. That isn't the way it works with most women. Some may still experience the classic symptom of heaviness in the chest, but women are more likely than men to experience atypical or less obvious symptoms. One thing to note: a heart attack is a form of heart disease, which is a broader term and can include other conditions that are not severe enough to cause a heart attack.

Heart *disease* symptoms may include the following:

- Pain in the jaw, teeth, neck, or back

- Upper abdominal pain: nausea, fullness, or a burning sensation in the abdomen or chest

- Shortness of breath either with exertion or at rest

- Excessive fatigue

- Palpitations (a sensation of fluttering in your chest)
- Fainting or lightheadedness

If you are experiencing any of these symptoms and they come on suddenly, seek immediate medical care. If they are intermittent and have been going on for weeks, see your physician as soon as possible. They could represent a blockage in a heart artery, a valve abnormality, a rhythm disturbance (excessively fast or slow beating of the heart), or heart failure (a disorder in which the heart muscle cannot pump effectively due to either inability to squeeze properly or to relax well). These symptoms may be caused by exertion, emotional distress, or no provocation whatsoever.

Heart *attack* symptoms may include the following:

- Sudden onset of pressure in the chest
- Lightheadedness
- Difficulty breathing
- Jaw pain, neck pain, or back pain associated with other cardiac symptoms

If you are experiencing any of these symptoms call 911—and be as proactive as you can be at the hospital. "Many women say, 'Oh, there's something not right with me,'" says health coach Donna Slicis, "where men are quicker to say, 'I'm dying. Help me.' Make the doctors and nurses feel as scared as you are."

Symptoms of *stroke* or *ministroke* may include the following:

- Loss of vision or double vision
- Difficulty speaking
- Weakness in an arm, leg, or both
- Severe headache along with one symptom

If you are experiencing any of these symptoms call 911 and, again, be forceful.

Risk Factors for Heart Disease

As I mentioned in chapter 1, in early 2011, the AHA released new guidelines for the prevention of cardiovascular disease in women. Included are updated guidelines for management of heart disease risk factors—those you can change and those you cannot, such as age, ethnicity, and family history. Following are the newest guidelines along with discussion of risk factors you can't change. I also talk about definite lifestyle and physiologic risk factors, as well as potential risk factors; these three categories are very much within your power to change.

You are at *high risk* for heart disease if you have one or more of the following conditions:

- Heart artery disease (you've suffered a heart attack, have a stent, or show blockage in your arteries)

- Blood vessel disease in the carotid arteries

- Prior stroke

- Plaque in the arteries of the abdomen or legs

- Abdominal aortic aneurysm (when the aorta or major blood vessel in the abdomen is dilated)

- End-stage or chronic kidney disease

- Diabetes

- Your ten-year predicted risk of cardiovascular disease is over 10 percent (something your health care provider can calculate for you using the Framingham Risk Score)

You are at *risk* for heart disease if you have one or more of the following:

- History of cigarette smoking
- Obesity, particularly an apple-shaped physique
- Physical inactivity
- Poor diet
- Family history of cardiovascular disease
- High blood pressure
- High cholesterol
- Metabolic syndrome, a series of symptoms that include a large waist circumference, high triglyceride level, low level of HDL (the "good" cholesterol), high blood pressure (also known as hypertension), and a high fasting glucose level
- History of preeclampsia, gestational diabetes, or high blood pressure associated with pregnancy
- Rheumatologic diseases, like lupus or rheumatoid arthritis
- Evidence of advanced atherosclerosis (thickening and hardening of the lining of the arteries of the body)
- Poor fitness level as indicated by a treadmill test, administered by a doctor, and/or abnormal heart rate recovery after stopping exercise

You are considered to be at *optimal risk* (the least amount of risk) if you have the following:

- Low total cholesterol, with optimal HDL cholesterol—the "good kind" (>50 mg/dl)
- Ideal blood pressure (<120/80 mmHg)

- Fasting blood glucose <100 mg/dl
- Body mass index <25 kg/m²
- Abstinence from smoking
- If you're over twenty years old and exercise 150 minutes/week at a moderate intensity, 75 minutes/week at a vigorous intensity—or do a combination of the two
- Consumption of a healthy diet, heavy on fruits and vegetables

Risk Factors Out of Your Control

While the following three categories are factors you cannot change, their presence is important to recognize because they do contribute to your overall heart risk.

Age

As with most things that get older—cars, wooden floors, your favorite pair of shoes—your heart shows signs of wear with age. Most notably, plaque builds up in the arteries of even the healthiest individuals. The heart muscle becomes less pliable and stiffens with age. The valves of the heart can also be damaged over time, leading to either narrowing or leakage. Although it's important to monitor the health of your heart at all ages, a turning point happens around age fifty-five for women, or roughly when menopause begins. For reasons still unclear to experts, estrogen, the hormone that drops precipitously during menopause, provides our hearts with some level of protection against disease. When that hormonal shield disappears, our hearts and circulatory systems have to fend for themselves—or, more accurately, you have to vigilantly take care of them, if you haven't already.

For now, there seems to be no medical solution for the absence of estrogen. The Women's Health Initiative, a comprehensive research program that involved 161,808 women and took place over fifteen years, concluded that the long-term use of hormone replacement therapy (estrogen plus progestin) in postmenopausal women increases the risk of heart attack, stroke, blood clots, and breast cancer.[1] The jury is still out when it comes to the potential beneficial effect of estrogen alone, or other preparations of estrogen. For now, it is off the table for heart disease prevention.

Family History

Your parents haven't just influenced your daily habits like how you eat, spend money, and vote; what happens or has happened in their bodies is likely to have a repeat performance in yours. Put more bluntly: if they had heart artery disease, you have an increased risk of having it too. Although your grandparents and aunts and uncles weigh in on your family medical tree, the biggest influence on your health is your *first-degree relatives*, or your parents and siblings. In fact, your risk goes up further if a first-degree relative contracted the disease before age sixty-five (if female) or age fifty-five (if male).

While devastating cardiac events, like heart attack and stroke, are linked to your genes, so are a number of other very important cardiac conditions. On the following pages is a comprehensive list of conditions and diseases that carry a genetic component. You should mention any of them to your physician at the time of an initial evaluation.

- *Atrial fibrillation*: Chaotic rhythm that occurs when the regular signal that starts the heartbeat is no longer present; instead, multiple signals bombard the heart at once, which leads to a rapid, irregular heart rhythm.

- *Bicuspid aortic valve*: an inherited condition in which the aortic valve is comprised of two leaflets instead of three

- Blood clots (especially important item for women who are considering starting or are on birth control pills)

- *Cardiomyopathy*, an abnormality of the heart muscle: it is not able to adequately pump and relax (or both) between heartbeats. A similar condition is *hypertrophic cardiomyopathy*, where the heart walls are excessively thick and dilated.

- Congenital narrowing of the aortic valve and other forms of congenital heart disease: a condition with which a person is born

- Diabetes

- Diseases that involve the aorta, or the major blood vessel of the body. Two common ones are an *aneurysm*, or the ballooning of the aorta, and *aortic dissection*, a condition in which the walls of the aorta split apart

- Heart attack

- Heart valve diseases, including *mitral valve prolapse*, a condition in which the upper and lower chambers of the left side of the heart do not close properly

- High blood pressure

- High cholesterol

- Marfan syndrome, a condition associated with excessive height, abnormalities of the eyes, bones, blood vessels, and heart: associated with an increased risk of aortic dissection

- Stroke
- Sudden cardiac death: An unexpected, quick death (less than an hour, usually, from onset of symptoms) due to cardiac causes in a person with known or unknown cardiac disease

If you are adopted, it is vitally important to find out your biological family's heart history. Adoption agencies are retaining more parental health records, so begin there—and if they can't help, ask if they have recommendations. If you're estranged from your biological parents, consider writing them a letter with simple questions or asking another blood relative to help complete a family medical tree.

Even if tracking down the information is complicated, the effort is well worth it. I recall the case of a seemingly healthy, fit, thirty-five-year-old woman who developed sudden intense pressure in her chest; she felt like she had an elephant parked on her breastbone. She called 911, and an ambulance came. Given that she was fit, a nonsmoker, and a nondiabetic on no medications, an EMT told her she was having a panic attack. She wasn't convinced he was correct.

Trusting her intuition, she insisted on a cardiac evaluation and was found to have a severe blockage in the main artery of her heart. In fact, she experienced cardiac arrest while undergoing the test. She was successfully resuscitated, underwent heart bypass surgery, and is healthy today.

The patient was adopted; after her heart attack, she found out that her birth father had had a very significant heart problem at a young age. Armed with this information, she will be able to provide her kids with their proper health history and hopefully prevent such devastating events in their lives.

That's the key about family history: even if your family seems to have more heart attacks than a thunderstorm has lightning strikes, realize that heart disease does not have to be your destiny. Armed with knowledge and willpower, you can change the course of your health—and that of the generations that follow you.

Ethnicity

Along with a physiological clock that only goes in one direction and a set of powerful genes, your ethnic background is also a key player in your risk for heart disease. Statistically, African-American and Latina women are at higher risk of developing heart artery disease and having a heart attack than white women. In a study from Duke University, doctors followed nearly twenty-three thousand patients with evidence of blockages in their heart arteries. After fifteen years, they found that African-American women had the lowest survival rates, while white men had the highest. The African-American patients were more likely to have diabetes, lower incomes, and heart failure, which may be part of the reason why they were the most likely to die.[2]

So out of the long list of risk factors on pages 36–37, there are only three things out of your control. All of the rest, no matter how daunting they may feel right now, are firmly within your grasp. In fact, many of them are interrelated: just like your overall life satisfaction is a web of many elements, no system in your body operates as a solo agent. If you lose weight, your blood pressure goes down, as do your cholesterol levels, and you've likely dropped pounds through exercise and modifying your diet. That's five risk factors tackled with one weight-loss bullet—I like that ratio. Let's start with discussing the lifestyle factors that matter most to your health.

Lifestyle Risk Factors

These are risk factors that are in your control; once you have recognized their presence, you can develop strategies to manage them.

Obesity

Turn on any channel, open any newspaper, surf the Internet regularly, and you'll see the obesity epidemic story popping up again and again. It truly is an epidemic. In the United States in 2009, only two places—Colorado and the District of Columbia—had a population with an obesity rate of less than 20 percent, according to the Centers for Disease Control and Prevention (CDC). Nine states clocked in with populations where at least one in three citizens are obese.[3] By obese, I don't mean carrying an extra twenty pounds. Obesity, by definition, is measured through *body mass index* (BMI), a ratio of weight to height squared, and is marked by a BMI equal to or greater than 30. A 5'8" person who weighs 200 pounds is obese, as is a 5'5" person who weighs 180 pounds. (Check your BMI at http://www.nhlbisupport.com/bmi/.)

Carrying extra pounds taxes your body—and heart—unnaturally. The more fat in a body, the more tiny the blood vessels, and the more the heart must pump to provide blood through these tiny vessels. Because the heart has to work harder, it eventually gets bigger—and weaker at the same time. It can slow the portion of the heartbeat during which the heart fills with blood, which makes you short of breath and raises blood pressure. Being overweight also causes a rise in blood pressure; one study found that women who are obese are three times as likely to have high blood pressure than those at a healthy weight.[4] And the extra calories that put on the pounds aren't likely to have been terribly healthy, which means cholesterol levels are probably an issue. Last but not least, contracting diabetes is also on the list of increased risk factors for obesity.

Smoking

Given all we know about how toxic cigarette smoking is, it continues to amaze me how many people smoke. "Smoking negates all the other good things going on in your body," says Kate Traynor, program director at the Cardiovascular Disease Prevention Center at Massachusetts General Hospital Heart Center. "All your numbers may be pristine—your cholesterol is on the money, your blood pressure is perfect, your weight is fine—but none of that matters if you smoke." Not surprisingly, cigarette smoking is the single most preventable cause of premature death in the United States. Not only is a smoker two to three times more likely to die from coronary heart disease than a nonsmoker is, but if you carry other risk factors and smoke, lighting up is basically a one-way ticket to your early funeral.[5] I realize that sounds harsh, but it's true.

Here's why: There is hardly a cell in the body that smoking doesn't affect. The chemicals from cigarettes speed up the formation of plaque on the walls of the coronary and other arteries. Nicotine causes blood vessels to constrict, which raises blood pressure and heart rate. Smoking reduces the amount of oxygen that gets distributed to your entire body and can lower the amount of HDL (good) cholesterol. What's more, if you need birth control, the pill isn't an option. Hormonally based contraception, combined with smoking, substantially increases your risk of developing blood clots or having a heart attack. Perhaps worse is secondhand smoke, which can cause heart attacks and lung cancer in nonsmoking adults; in children, it has been linked to sudden infant death syndrome, respiratory infections, and middle-ear infections, among other things.

I have talked to enough patients who are smokers to know that quitting is difficult. The sidebar below gives you some effective strategies; even if you've tried to quit numerous times, it's worth another shot. Cardiovascular risk starts to decrease the day you put down the cigarettes, and within five to fifteen years of being smoke-free your risk is equal to that of a nonsmoker. In addition to lowering your heart disease risk by stopping smoking, you also lower your risk of several forms of cancer, lung disease, and disease in the blood vessels throughout the body.

Kick the Butts Forever

Although I've never been a smoker, I am fully aware of how difficult it is to quit the habit. Still, stopping smoking is the single most beneficial health choice you can make for your physical health and overall well-being. Researchers from the United Kingdom found that quitting smoking is associated with increased happiness. Polling 879 ex-smokers, almost 70 percent reported being happier now than they were when they were smoking, while only 3 percent were less happy. (Given that many smokers rely on cigarettes for emotional support, this is an unexpected and helpful finding.) One caveat the scientists found was that greater happiness was associated with having quit more than a year ago, so patience is rewarded.[6]

Here, Susan Lane, who leads smoking cessation programs through the Massachusetts General Hospital system, shares some strategies that have worked for people in her classes.

- **Get some support.** Many community and health centers have smoking cessation programs; as HAPPY Heart has shown, it's invaluable to talk to other people who are experiencing the same thing you are.

- **Try not to puff your way out of stress anymore.** "The answer I hear almost constantly when I ask why someone smokes is stress," says Lane. "The best way to rid yourself of stress is exercise: it clears your mind and energizes your body." She recommends you start walking or doing other easy exercise before you even try to stop smoking. That way, when you do begin to quit, you'll have another option for stress release.

- **Don't go cold turkey.** Instead, Lane has her students decrease their cigarette intake one at a time. "Go from thirty cigarettes to twenty-nine cigarettes for a week," she says. "Make it so small that it feels achievable." There's another reason for the minimal decrease: if you go too quickly, the nicotine receptors in your brain feel the deprivation and make you want to smoke even more. A gradual decrease keeps them quiet.

- **When you do go slowly, realize that it may take at least six weeks, and could take as long as six months.** "Congratulate yourself every time you succeed at eliminating another cigarette," she says. "That's a great step in the right direction."

- **Hold your nose when you smoke.** "You'll get zero pleasure out of the cigarette," says Lane. "It makes it tasteless."

- **When you smoke, only smoke.** Don't check your email, drink coffee, drive your car, or chat with a friend. Concentrate only on that cigarette. "So often we associate smoking with another behavior," she says, "so you're not even cognizant of the cigarette. This makes you very aware of it."

- **When you're concentrating on that cigarette, get out of your physical comfort zone.** Stand when you smoke (or, better yet, stand on one foot) or sit in a hard-backed chair. "Nothing smoking-related should be comfortable."

- **When you do succeed at quitting, realize that you might feel depressed and/or anxious.** "So many smokers think of cigarettes as their best friends, and not having that relationship anymore can be really hard," says Lane. Be in conversation with your primary care doctor; therapy or short-term medication for depression might be good options.

Physiological Risk Factors

Knowledge about the following risk factors, or "knowing your numbers," gives you the power to address them. Your medical provider should have most of the pertinent numerical information, but if you have not seen her recently, then you should schedule an appointment to get your updated numbers.

High Blood Pressure

Often called the silent killer, high blood pressure (*hypertension* or HBP) is extremely dangerous because it lurks in your body and exhibits very few outward symptoms. In fact, the only sure way to know if you have hypertension is to measure your blood pressure (BP). The initial diagnosis requires multiple readings. Several will be taken in your doctor's office, but it is also important to keep an eye on your BP at home if your readings have been borderline or high.

The silence of high blood pressure can be deadly though; it increases your chance of a heart attack, heart failure, stroke, kidney disease, and blood vessel disease, including aortic dissection and peripheral blood vessel disease. Even when it is diagnosed, it can be a stubborn disease. Of the 70 percent of people with hypertension who are being treated, a full 53 percent still do not have their blood pressure under control.[7]

What's more mystifying about high blood pressure is that the specific cause of 90 to 95 percent of the cases of high blood pressure isn't known.[8] While it's more common in people who exhibit other risk factors for cardiovascular disease and is often associated with unhealthy lifestyle habits, I still can't look at a person and know with certainty if they have it. For example, I have one patient who works out regularly, weighs 128 pounds, and is basically the picture of health, except for her blood pressure. After menopause, her body changed radically, and her blood pressure can now get up to a dangerous level of 190/100.

The basics of blood pressure are well known though. Blood pressure results from the combination of blood being pumped out of the heart and the resistance provided by the blood vessels. It is influenced by three aspects of the circulatory system: the force of the heart's contraction, the tone of the *arterioles* (the body's smallest arteries) and their ability to widen or narrow, and the volume of blood moving through the system. The kidneys, which secrete chemicals that direct how the blood vessels respond to pressure, are essentially the control panel for blood pressure.

A blood pressure reading is given as two numbers, with one over the other (for example, 120/80). The *systolic number* (on top) measures the pressure generated against the arterial walls when the heart pumps. The *diastolic pressure* (on the bottom) measures the pressure in the vessels when the heart is relaxed.

Some Surprising Causes of High Blood Pressure

- **Preeclampsia.** Pregnant women who experienced *preeclampsia* (a condition marked by high blood pressure, leg swelling, and protein in the urine after twenty weeks gestation) have been found to be more likely to develop high blood pressure postpregnancy. Women who have preeclampsia likely already have—but may not know they have—blood vessels that don't relax appropriately. Because pregnancy stresses the body, it magnifies previously unknown issues, so the preeclampsia diagnosis can actually be a tip-off that a woman needs to carefully watch her blood pressure in the future.

- **Coarctation of the aorta.** A discrete narrowing in the aorta on the left side of the body, coarctation of the aorta is a form of heart disease a person is born with. The condition reduces blood flow to the kidneys, resulting in high blood pressure.

- **Low birth weight.** A birth weight below 2.6 pounds (1,250 grams [g]) puts a person at high risk for high blood pressure. Kidneys are the command center for blood pressure and mature very rapidly in the last four to eight weeks in utero. If a baby is born before thirty-two weeks, which is typical for a baby with low birth weight, the kidneys are likely not fully developed and don't function optimally.

- **Birth control pills.** Oral contraceptives can increase blood pressure in some women, especially if they are overweight or have had high blood pressure during pregnancy, a family history of HBP, or mild kidney disease. Before you go on the pill, make sure your doctor records your blood pressure and that you have it checked every six months or so.

Also, be sure you thoroughly discuss your family's health history, especially with regard to blood clotting. Paige, a patient and close friend of mine, is a great athlete and incredibly fit. At forty-six and approaching menopause, she went on the pill, as many women do, to make the transition smoother. Her doctor didn't ask about her family history; her mother had died at age twenty-nine from a blood clot in her lung. Paige called me one day and mentioned her calf was really sore. I asked if she had been running a lot or otherwise taxed it, and she answered no; she and her husband actually had recently been on a trip to Australia. Knowing the relationship between flying and the risk of blood clots, I told her to get to the emergency room as soon as possible. She was lucky: her entire leg was filled with clots, and if they had broken off and traveled to her lungs, the story could have ended tragically.

HOW IS BLOOD PRESSURE DIAGNOSED?

Blood pressure is most commonly taken with a blood pressure cuff in a medical office. Healthy blood pressure is considered to be less than 120/80. *Prehypertension*, a condition that doubles your risk of hypertension, is diagnosed when the systolic number is between 120 to 139 or the diastolic number is between 80 to 89. Hypertension occurs when blood pressure is greater than 140/90 on a regular basis. If you have a high reading, you should have two or more readings over a period of one to three weeks to confirm.

HOW OFTEN SHOULD BLOOD PRESSURE BE MEASURED?

If your numbers are 120/80 or less, current guidelines recommend blood pressure screening every two years. People with prehypertension should have their blood pressure checked annually, at a minimum.

If you have high blood pressure, your doctor will likely advise you to get a home blood pressure monitoring unit that you can use to measure and keep track of your blood pressure at home. The basic units run under eighty dollars and are easy to use. When a patient of mine is either starting medication to control hypertension or adjusting her dose, I ask her to take her pressure every other day, in the morning and at night, until we can see the results of the change. She can write down her numbers on a sheet of paper and then log them on a computer or use an iPhone app, which is useful because it graphs the highs and lows. Once we figure out the correct dosage, she can be less vigilant about home monitoring.

Know Your Numbers

Even if you have healthy blood pressure, it's never a bad idea to check it when you have a chance:

- Use the blood pressure machines available in pharmacies.
- Many dentists now check blood pressure, as do gynecologists.
- If you have a nurse in your office, ask her to check yours when she has some downtime.
- Get it checked at a health fair at a mall.

WHO IS AT RISK FOR HIGH BLOOD PRESSURE?

A better question might be, who isn't at risk? According to the Centers for Disease Control and Prevention, 74.5 million Americans have hypertension—or one in three adults. In addition, 25 percent of American adults have prehypertension. Before age fifty, hypertension is more common in men than in women. But as we females age, we make up ground quickly; from age fifty-five on, we dominate the cases, according to the CDC. By age seventy-five, the CDC reports that 65 percent of men and 80 percent of women will be diagnosed with high blood pressure.[9]

Age is one risk factor for hypertension, as is genetics. If you have a family history of high blood pressure or heart disease, you're at a significantly greater risk to contract it. Finally, be aware that African-Americans develop high blood pressure more often, and at an earlier age, than other ethnic groups. These factors are obviously out of your control.

What can you control? Plenty. Other proven risk factors include an unhealthy weight, high cholesterol levels, lack of exercise, drinking more than two alcoholic drinks daily, and a diet that is high in fat and salt. (There's a reason why those drive-through fries taste so good; they're coated in salt. In fact, researchers at the Center for Science in the Public Interest analyzed 102 meals from seventeen popular chain restaurants and found that 85 of them had 1,500 milligrams (mg) more than the daily recommendation of sodium. Some had as much as four days' worth.[10]) Science hasn't uncovered solid proof that smoking, stress, and sleep apnea are definitive risk factors, but there seems to be a strong association.

HOW IS HIGH BLOOD PRESSURE TREATED?
Treatment depends on the severity of the measurements. Lifestyle adaptations—reducing salt in the diet, exercising, quitting smoking, losing weight—are always recommended for anybody with higher than normal numbers. Behavior modifications are usually the starting point for people with prehypertension, and if the blood pressure doesn't respond accordingly, medication will likely be started.

Typically, if the measurement is 140/90 or above, or 130/80 in somebody who has kidney disease or diabetes, medication is prescribed, along with lifestyle changes.

BLOOD PRESSURE MEDICATIONS

DRUG	WHAT IT DOES	SIDE EFFECTS/ CAUTIONS	RECOMMENDED FOR
Diuretic	• Increases removal of sodium through the kidneys. • Decreases blood volume.	• Potassium supplementation (either through an oral supplement or daily banana, orange, or tomato juice) required for the nonpotassium-sparing diuretics. • May lower potassium and magnesium and raise blood glucose and cholesterol levels. • Diuretics may raise triglyceride levels in the blood.	• Most women, unless their health history conflicts with their use.
ACE inhibitors: Angiotensin converting enzyme inhibitors	• Reduces constriction of blood vessels by blocking the formation of angiotensin II and formation of aldosterone.	• A dry hacking cough (3%–35% of patients are affected by this); can cause dangerously high potassium levels in the presence of abnormal kidney function.	• Women with history of coronary artery disease or heart attack. • **Should not be used by pregnant women.**
ARBs: Angiotensin receptor blockers	• Interferes with binding of angiotensin II to its receptor, resulting in a decrease in blood vessel resistance and blood pressure.	• Fewer side effects than ACE inhibitors. • Increased potassium levels can be an issue.	• Women with history of coronary artery disease or heart attack. • **Should not be used by pregnant women.**
Calcium channel blockers	• Relaxes some of the blood vessels. • Lowers blood pressure. • They may also reduce symptoms of angina or chest pain.	• Some may slow heart rate slightly, cause swelling in the ankles, headaches, and flushing (becoming red in the face).	• Women for whom other agents have not been effective. • Women with a history of heart artery disease.

Hypertension by Any Other Name

When a patient has elevated blood pressure in the doctor's office but has normal numbers at home, it's referred to as *white-coat hypertension*; it is present in as many as one in three of patients. It was originally thought to be a benign condition stemming from the jitters related to potentially receiving bad news or a painful injection, but recent data suggests that there is nothing benign about it. In 2010, investigators from Spain compared the heart ultrasounds of individuals with normal blood pressure, white-coat hypertension, and high blood pressure. Looking at left ventricular hypertrophy, or abnormally thick hearts that result from strenuously working to pump blood, 13.2 percent of the patients with normal pressure had the condition, compared to 49.1 percent with white-coat hypertension and 54.3 percent of the hypertensive patients. "The implications [of white-coat hypertension] are closer to those of sustained hypertension than to those of normal blood pressure," they conclude.[11]

The opposite of white-coat hypertension, *masked hypertension* occurs when the blood pressure readings in the doctor's office are normal but are elevated during day-to-day monitoring. This can occur due to the hectic, stressful, adrenaline-stimulating lives of some who, when confronted with a calm, quiet doctor's office, suddenly become very relaxed. Just like white-coat hypertension, masked hypertension is surprisingly dangerous; a group of investigators from Italy followed 1,412 people for ten years. At the first measuring, 124 of the patients had masked hypertension. A decade later, nearly half—fifty-six—of the cases of masked hypertension had morphed into high blood pressure.[12] If you or your doctor suspects you could have masked hypertension, your physician should consider ordering a twenty-four-hour ambulatory blood pressure monitor.

High Cholesterol

Cholesterol is another important buzzword around heart health. Cholesterol is a waxy, fatty substance integral to many of the body's functions. It is needed to make vitamin D, some hormones, bile acids that aid in fat digestion, and the walls of all the body's cells.

Cholesterol gets into the body in two ways: The liver makes about 1000 milligrams of it daily. How the liver processes that cholesterol is largely up to genetics; based on one's genes, it can go into the bloodstream and either integrate itself into arteries (not good) or end up in the liver (good), where the body excretes it. (Note: The liver produces enough cholesterol for your body without needing supplementation.) The second way cholesterol can get into the body, you already know: food. Animal-based foods such as meat, eggs, and dairy products contain cholesterol. By restricting saturated fat (fats that are found in animal products, as well as coconut and palm oils) and cholesterol-heavy foods (the list includes animal organs (like liver), ice cream, and cheese), you can give your liver less material to work with. Reducing cholesterol in your diet can result in as much as a 10 percent reduction in your overall levels.

Cholesterol is a *lipid* (a fat). Fats can't travel alone through the body, so certain proteins attach to the cholesterol and form a molecule made up of fat and protein—a *lipoprotein*. There are six lipoprotein measurements that can be considered when monitoring cholesterol levels in the blood:

1. **Low-density lipoprotein (LDL—the bad kind of cholesterol).** Directly associated with an increased risk of heart disease, LDL is linked to atherosclerosis, the buildup of plaque that hardens the arteries and increases your risk of coronary heart disease and heart attack.

2. **High-density lipoprotein (HDL—the good kind of choles-terol).** The opposite of LDL, HDL particles clear out the LDL particles, reducing the level of plaque and lowering the risk for coronary artery disease. They transport cholesterol back to the liver, where it is excreted by the body.

3. **Triglycerides.** The most common kind of fat in the body, triglycerides are actually used for energy. When your body doesn't need all the calories you eat, the surplus are stored as triglycerides and carried in the blood as *very-low-density lipoprotein* (VLDL). While elevated triglycerides are linked to the development of atherosclerosis, the connection is nowhere near as strong as that of LDL cholesterol and atherosclerosis.

4. **Non-HDL cholesterol.** This is the total cholesterol level minus the HDL level. This number accurately predicts future heart events in women and appears to be better at prediction of these events than measurement of specific lipoproteins.

5. **Lipoprotein-associated phospholipase A2 (Lp-PLA).** This measurement reflects the interaction between inflammation and lipid processing. It is produced as part of the inflamma-tory reaction (a body's attempt to repair itself; it is usually associated with production of white blood cells and the heal-ing chemicals they release) and is attached to LDL cholesterol. Although it predicts future heart events regardless of other risk factors, it has not yet been incorporated into management guidelines.

6. **Lipoprotein (a), apolipoprotein B, and small dense LDL.** These three lipoproteins also correlate with heart risk and are often measured in individuals who have a family history of heart disease affecting people at a young age. These lipids are often targets of treatment after the LDL and HDL goals are met.

HOW IS HIGH CHOLESTEROL DIAGNOSED?

The National Cholesterol Education Program recommends that adults twenty years of age or older have a fasting cholesterol profile completed every five years. The test, a simple blood draw, requires you to fast (no food, liquids, or pills) for nine to twelve hours. Your doctor may choose to follow less rigorous guidelines and start with a nonfasting test if you have no risk factors, and then commence the fasting tests in men over thirty-five and women over forty-five. If the opposite is true—you have risk factors or your cholesterol levels are borderline or elevated—your doctor will likely opt to check your levels more frequently.

CHOLESTEROL TEST RESULTS AND WHAT THEY MEAN
(ACCORDING TO THE AMERICAN HEART ASSOCIATION)

	MEASUREMENT	DIAGNOSIS
Total cholesterol	Less than 200 mg/dl	Normal
	200–239 mg/dl	Borderline high
	240 mg/dl and above	• High blood cholesterol • Risk of coronary heart disease is twice that of somebody with normal levels
LDL (bad) cholesterol	Less than 100 mg/dl	Optimal
	100–129 mg/dl	Near or above optimal
	130–159 mg/dl	Borderline high
	160–189 mg/dl	High
	190 mg/dl and above	Very high
HDL (good) cholesterol	Less than 50 mg/dl for women (for men, less than 40 mg/dl)	Low; a major risk factor for heart disease
	60 mg/dl and above	Optimal; considered protective against heart disease

	MEASUREMENT	DIAGNOSIS
Triglycerides	Less than 150 mg/dl	Normal
	150–199 mg/dl	Borderline high
	200–499 mg/dl	High
	500 mg/dl and above	Very high
Non-HDL cholesterol* (Total cholesterol – HDL)	<130 mg/dl	Normal

* This is a helpful number to know, because it separates the good from the bad; if a woman's HDL is 80 mg/dl, her overall number may seem high but actually isn't as bad as it sounds.

WHO IS AT RISK FOR HIGH CHOLESTEROL?

As with most risk factors, cholesterol is a combination of factors within and outside of your control. Within your control are the usual suspects: eating a nutritious diet low in saturated fats, keeping your weight in a healthy range, not smoking, exercising regularly. Age—men aged forty-five years and older and women aged fifty-five and older—increases the risk of high cholesterol, as does gender. Estrogen raises HDL levels, so when menopause occurs and estrogen levels plummet, a woman's LDL level tends to rise. Family history again plays a role: if your immediate family was affected by high cholesterol, there's a decent chance you will be too.

HOW IS CHOLESTEROL TREATED?

As you might expect, the initial treatment for high cholesterol is to make lifestyle changes. A great place to start, if appropriate, is quitting smoking; smoking lowers HDL cholesterol levels and increases the tendency for blood to clot. Dietary changes also help; even though the body produces all the cholesterol it needs, the average American eats over 200 milligrams a day, which is what the AHA recommends for people with coronary heart disease.[13] Since foods from animals are the primary source of cholesterol, the AHA recommends no more than six ounces of lean meat, fish, or poultry daily, and to eat either low-fat or fat-free dairy products. Finally, exercise is an easy way to get your numbers under control; regular exercise reduces the amount of LDL and increases the amount of HDL.

If you have an increased risk of heart disease, conditions like diabetes or kidney disease, or an LDL level higher than 190 mg/dl, your doctor will likely suggest that you complement your lifestyle changes with a medication.

COMMON DRUGS USED TO TREAT CHOLESTEROL

DRUG	WHAT IT DOES	SIDE EFFECTS	RECOMMENDED FOR
Statins	• Reduces level of LDL and VLDL. • Also decreases C-reactive protein and inflammation. • Also proven to prevent heart attacks and strokes in women.	• Muscle pain or weakness. • Elevated levels on muscle enzymes and liver function tests.	• Women with established coronary artery or vascular disease or diabetes. • Those at high risk for cardiovascular disease.
Fibrates	• Lowers LDL and triglycerides. • Raises HDL. • May prevent a second cardiac event in individuals with low HDL levels.	• Abdominal discomfort. • Liver function abnormalities. • Skin rash. • Interaction with other medications. • Possible interference with statins, increasing the likelihood of muscle aches and weakness.	• Individuals with metabolic syndrome who have low HDL (<50 mg/dl) and high triglycerides (>150 mg/dl). • Also high-risk women after LDL goal is reached.

DRUG	WHAT IT DOES	SIDE EFFECTS	RECOMMENDED FOR
Niacin	• Increases HDL levels and lowers triglycerides. • Does *not* lower LDL.	• Flushing (redness in the face), reduced by taking daily aspirin. • Elevated levels of uric acid and blood glucose. • Liver and gastrointestinal (GI) side effects.	• Individuals with metabolic syndrome.
Fish oil	• Decreases formation of VLDL. • In large doses (up to 10 g/day), may lower triglycerides.	• Aftertaste. • Slightly increased risk of bleeding.	• Everyone.

Diabetes

Our body's cells need sugar, also known as *glucose*, to function; glucose provides the body with energy. For the glucose to move into cells and be processed, insulin, a hormone produced by the pancreas, is needed. Diabetes occurs when there isn't enough insulin in the body for the glucose to get into the cells, and, as a result, levels of blood sugars rise.

Diabetes is a chronic disease. There are two types:

- Type 1 is usually diagnosed in childhood and makes up 5 percent of the diabetes cases nationwide, according to the American Diabetes Association (ADA). In this type of diabetes, the pancreas makes little or no insulin.

- Type 2 is far more common and diagnosed in all ages. It occurs when the body does not produce enough insulin or the cells ignore the insulin available.

Although diabetes can't be cured, it can be controlled, and it needs to be for a variety of reasons. Diabetes alone is one of the symptoms in the high-risk category for cardiovascular disease; the association is so strong that many diabetics are treated as if they have heart disease. According to the ADA, people with diabetes have heart disease death rates and stroke risks that are two to four times higher than adults without diabetes.[14] Not surprisingly, diabetes also has a strong association with high blood pressure; the ADA reports that from 2005 to 2008, 67 percent of American adults with diabetes had blood pressure greater than or equal to 140/90 or used prescription medications for hypertension.[15] Left untreated, diabetes damages small blood vessels and may cause kidney disease, nervous system damage, blindness, and even result in amputation of the limbs.

HOW IS DIABETES DIAGNOSED?

Although diabetes, particularly type 2, can often have no symptoms, there are a few warning signs: excessive thirst, frequent urination and infections, fatigue, blurred vision, and tingling in the hands and feet.

Diabetes is diagnosed via a few markers that measure the level of glucose in the blood. If everyday blood glucose levels are greater than or equal to 200 mg/dl, there's a strong possibility that a person has diabetes. Some additional tests confirm a diagnosis:

- **A fasting blood glucose test** requires that you don't eat or drink anything with calories for eight to twelve hours prior to the test. If these levels are greater than 126 mg/dl, diabetes is diagnosed. (Normal fasting blood glucose level is less than or equal to 100 mg/dl.)

- **The hemoglobin A1C** is frequently checked. It reflects glucose levels over the past two to three months. Normal levels are 4 to 6 percent, and a level greater than 6.5 percent indicates diabetes.

- **A glucose tolerance test,** during which you drink a highly sweetened beverage and have your glucose levels tested, is one more diagnostic tool. If glucose levels are greater than 200 mg/dl two hours after the test, this also indicates diabetes.

You're not in the clear if your numbers don't match any of these numbers. Impaired glucose tolerance is a condition in which the glucose levels come back slightly lower than the ones cited in the previous paragraph (fasting glucose: 100–125 mg/dl; hemoglobin A1C: 5.7 to 6.4 percent; glucose tolerance test: 140–199 mg/dl two hours after test). These numbers are cause for serious concern, as they also increase the risk of heart disease.

WHO IS AT RISK FOR DIABETES?

Too many people: According to statistics released by the CDC in early 2011, 25.8 million children and adults in the United States—8.3 percent of the population—have it. What's more, 78 million people have *prediabetes*, which frequently leads to diabetes.[16]

Since most type 1 diabetes cases are diagnosed in childhood, type 2 is the focus for our purposes. Obesity is a major risk factor, and as average weights go up, so does the prevalence of diabetes. In fact, as I mentioned earlier, due to this strong connection, a new term has been coined by medical professionals to describe the oncoming epidemic: "diabesity." According to CDC data, every baby born in or after 2000 has a one-in-three chance of becoming a diabetic, and female Hispanic and African-American children are at the highest risk with about one in two being at risk of developing diabetes.[17]

If you developed gestational diabetes during pregnancy, research shows that you have a one-in-three chance of becoming a diabetic.

Finally, people sixty-five and older are also at increased risk: over one in four in this age group is a diabetic.[18]

HOW IS DIABETES TREATED?

It depends on the type. Diabetics with type 1 simply don't have enough insulin on board, so they either inject themselves with the hormone or have a pump placed under the skin that releases insulin as needed.

Many people with type 2 also need to take insulin, either as a standing dose or less frequently to maintain a desirable glucose level. Type 2 diabetics may also take other medications that help lower blood glucose levels. More importantly, diet and nutrition—the two keys to getting to and maintaining a healthy weight—are huge. The Diabetes Prevention Program, a major multicenter research study that involved 3,234 people with prediabetes, compared the results of a lifestyle change (healthy eating and physical activity) with that of taking the diabetes drug metformin. The group that exercised thirty minutes a day, five days a week, usually by walking, and lowered their fat and overall caloric intake, lost an average of fifteen pounds in the first year and lowered their risk of getting type 2 diabetes by 58 percent. (Even more promising were the results for those aged sixty and older, who reduced their risk by 71 percent.) In comparison, those on the drug lowered their risk by 31 percent.[19]

Metabolic Syndrome

Metabolic syndrome is a combination of physical symptoms that exist when someone has three of the following five risk factors:

- Large waist circumference (greater than or equal to 35 inches in women; greater than 40 inches in men)

- High triglyceride level (greater than or equal to 150 mg/dl)

- Low HDL cholesterol level (less than 50 mg/dl in women; less than 45 mg/dl in men)

- Elevated blood pressure (greater than 130/85 mmHg)

- High fasting glucose level (greater than 100 mg/dl)

WHAT ARE THE RISKS OF METABOLIC SYNDROME?

Because so many of the factors of metabolic syndrome overlap with cardiovascular risk factors, the syndrome is associated with a greater risk of heart disease (two to three times higher than the risk in individuals without metabolic syndrome) and diabetes (four to ten times higher) as well as a greater likelihood of developing fatty liver disease and reproductive disorders.

Although the syndrome is well recognized by the cardiology community, I was worried that this association may not have been understood as well by primary care providers. While primary care physicians have learned to address breast and cervical cancer prevention in an efficient and systematic way, the same approach has not yet been taken with regard to women's heart health, especially when it comes to metabolic syndrome. It has been flying under the radar of many primary care physicians because they were not aware of how to diagnose it, didn't even know they needed to diagnose it, or simply did not realize how common it is—and how important it is to recognize it when it appears. So my HAPPY Heart team and I decided to determine how common metabolic syndrome was among the women in our study and how many actually had been diagnosed with it prior to entering the program. We found that 62.7 percent of the women in HAPPY Heart met the criteria for metabolic syndrome, yet only 2 percent were officially diagnosed with it prior to entering the study. Clearly, this syndrome is not at the forefront of well-known diseases, either for primary care physicians or for the majority of women, so it's essential if you're reading this book to equip yourself with knowledge; bring this up with your provider if you fit the metabolic syndrome symptoms.

If you think you may have metabolic syndrome, it is vital that you mention your concerns to your doctor, as more serious diseases will likely result from it. Although it may be hard to stomach, being diagnosed with metabolic syndrome is a wake-up call that can be answered with your own power. Often, it can be successfully treated with lifestyle modifications.

Potential Risk Factors for Heart Disease

Even though the AHA doesn't formally recognize the following categories as definitive risk factors for heart disease, the scientific evidence for including them is mounting.

Stress

Many people live today with a BlackBerry in one hand and a to-do list in another—and that's just for work. Add in all the other issues that can raise the hair on the back of your neck—everything from an unexpectedly long commute to a fight with your partner to a 401(k) account that isn't as robust as you thought it would be at this point— and it's no wonder that when asked, "How are you?" you respond with the twenty-first-century catchword: "Stressed."

Unfortunately, stress isn't just a state of mind. It can wreak havoc on your body and heart. When you feel stressed, your body transforms into fight-or-flight mode, which is its way of protecting you from potential danger. When you're hit with a sudden deadline, your credit card gets declined, or you hear some troubling news about a family member, the adrenal glands secrete hormones, like adrenaline, noradrenaline, and cortisol; the hormones basically prepare the troops for action. Your heart rate and blood pressure increase; the level of glucose, or easily accessible energy, rises in your blood; your muscles tense so you can either run or fight back.

Problem is, it's hard to fight a menacing BlackBerry. So your body has become agitated, and there isn't an easy way to diffuse the stress. The BlackBerry and to-do lists and rough times in a relationship will always be there, and they take a toll. Some people are able to handle a higher level of stress than others, while some crumble when they initially begin to feel overwhelmed.

Similarly, bodies react differently to levels of stress. We do know that chronically high stress levels can touch nearly every aspect of the body, causing everything from headaches to upset stomachs to fertility problems. When it comes to the heart, stress can wreak havoc, both directly and indirectly. Chronic stress levels lead to elevated levels of cortisol, which can, over time, keep your blood pressure and heart rate elevated and change, in an unfavorable way, how you metabolize sugar and fat. Stress can also lead to inactivity, consumption of fatty foods, excessive drinking, irregularly taking medications, and increased smoking, if you are a smoker. Finally, the detrimental effect of stress on sleep can also have a harmful impact on your health.

Alcohol Use

While the good news about red wine made media headlines—a handful of recent studies showed that moderate consumption can lower your risk of death from heart disease—it doesn't follow with red wine, or any other alcohol for that matter, that if some is good, more is better.[20] Excessive alcohol consumption, defined by the newest guidelines as more than one 12-ounce drink daily, can lead to high blood pressure, high triglycerides, and liver problems, among other things. New research, published in early 2011, studied the association of cancer and alcohol consumption in over 360,000 people in eight European countries and found that drinking predicted 10 percent of the cancer cases in men and 3 percent of them in women; drinking above the daily upper limits (European standards are 24 grams for men and 12 grams for women) substantially increased the risk of cancer.[21]

Although many people use a drink to take the edge off a stressful day, drinking can actually make stress worse. Because alcohol is dehydrating, the loss of water that occurs when you drink can cause the body to produce cortisol, the hormone described above that is associated with stress.

Alcohol is also such a powerful substance; people who have problems with excessive consumption are often so dependent on drinking that they frequently are unable to put their health first. At the Cardiovascular Disease Prevention Center at MGH, there are various disease-prevention groups that meet; participants complete self-evaluations before a new session begins. One is the CAGE questionnaire, a four-question screening test for alcohol dependence. Here are the questions:

- Have you ever felt you should cut down on your drinking?

- Have people annoyed you by criticizing your drinking?

- Have you ever felt bad or guilty about your drinking?

- Have you ever had a drink first thing in the morning to steady your nerves or get rid of a hangover (eye-opener)?

"If someone answers yes to two of those questions, there's a high chance she'll drop out of the program," says Traynor, the program director. "It's a pattern we've seen repeatedly."

Finally, even if drinking isn't a behavioral issue with you, it's worth remembering that alcohol can contribute to serious weight gain. I remember a patient who came to see me because her father had his first heart attack when he was only thirty-eight years old. At forty-four years old, she was in better health than her father, but she was still forty pounds overweight and had high blood pressure and high cholesterol. When we discussed her habits, she mentioned she drank three to four glasses of wine nightly with her husband. Doing some quick math, we calculated that by giving up the nightly wine she could save herself nearly six thousand calories a week. Surprised by that number, she corked her wine drinking, started exercising and eating better, and lost those extra forty pounds in only four months, getting her blood pressure under control in the meantime.

C-Reactive Protein

C-reactive protein (CRP) is a protein in the blood. Levels are increased in the presence of inflammatory conditions (arthritis, lupus) and infections.

WHAT ARE THE RISKS OF C-REACTIVE PROTEIN?

There is a great deal of controversy in the medical literature about the role of CRP in predicting cardiovascular risk. While the data clearly shows that the higher levels of CRP often correlate with heart disease, it is not clear whether CRP is merely a sign of cardiovascular disease or if it actually plays a role in causing heart problems. Part of the puzzle is that inflammatory disorders are, on their own, associated with an increased risk of heart disease. But when C-reactive protein is elevated in the absence of other obvious health problems, it may be an ominous predictor of heart disease risk. CRP levels may be more telling in women than in men, and can, if necessary, be lowered by using statins.

Diseases Linked to Heart Disease

Unfortunately, like diabetes, which is discussed on page 60, sometimes one diagnosis of a serious disease inherently carries with it an increased risk for heart disease. Here are two more to be aware of:

- **Breast cancer.** Many of the treatments for breast cancer have detrimental cardiovascular effects, including chemotherapeutic agents and radiation therapy, both of which can cause the heart muscle to weaken over time. Treatments can also bring on premature menopause, which means protective estrogen is gone, not to mention the stress associated with a devastating illness with major health impacts. Physicians from Duke University investigated the links in a study, and concluded that lifestyle changes are vital as a preemptive strike against the risk of heart disease.[22]

- **Rheumatologic diseases.** Diseases such as rheumatoid arthritis and lupus are more likely to occur in women, and the number one cause of death in women who are diagnosed with either disease is heart attack. Because the inflammatory conditions accelerate the formation of arterial plaque and blood clots, there is an excessive risk for heart attack, congestive heart failure, and stroke. Of particular concern are women in the thirty-five to forty-four age group, because heart disease is rare in young women, and they have a higher risk of a more severe outcome than their older counterparts.

Although I've given you general guidelines in this chapter to improve your physical health risk factors, the following chapters will go in depth into how to manage stress, eat better, motivate yourself to exercise, and consider the other parts of your life that influence your health.

Three Easy First Steps Across the Physical Health Bridge

1. **Grow a tree.** If you haven't yet, investigate and document your family health history. Share it with your siblings and children.

2. **Know your numbers.** If it's been more than two years since you've seen a primary care doctor, make an appointment today. Leave that appointment making sure you know your numbers, which include blood pressure, body mass index, fasting glucose level, and cholesterol. (You should have a fasting panel, which charts HDL, LDL, triglycerides, and total cholesterol, if it has been more than five years since you had one done, you have heart disease risk, or you have had abnormal results in the past.)

3. **Think about drink.** If you drink, evaluate your use of alcohol. Do you drink more than one serving daily? If so, consider slowly decreasing the amount consumed until you reach the recommended amount of no more than one drink per day (or better yet, reduce it further so you're drinking less than seven drinks weekly).

chapter three

The Emotional Health Bridge

Think about a typical day and the range of emotions you might go through. Maybe you wake up and feel annoyed when you realize your teenage son has finished off the milk—black coffee for you this morning. Then you head to work, and there's an accident that turns your fifteen-minute commute into forty-five minutes. You're a little irritated and feeling panicked because you were counting on that time to finish a presentation. You're stressed moments before you start the presentation, then elated when, upon finishing it, your boss gives you a thumbs-up. You go to lunch with a coworker, who tells you about her marital problems, and you have sympathy for her. The rest of the day is a cruise, until you get home, hungry and exhausted, and pick a fight with your husband because, well, you're hungry and exhausted and he hasn't started dinner like he promised he would. He makes amends by doing the dishes, letting you watch your favorite TV show, and coming to cuddle with you on the couch after he's done. The day ends with you feeling content and loved.

We often say, you are what you eat. That's mostly true, but I think this statement is much more accurate: you are what you feel. Through each of those everyday scenarios, your body reacted to what your mind was thinking. Different feelings can release hormones, speed up your heart rate and blood pressure, activate various areas of your brain, and otherwise turn into a catalyst for other physiological responses. For too many years, the medical community failed to consider that emotions carry such physiological weight and that they might be as integral to your health as more tangible contributors.

It's not that the emotional connection didn't cross anyone's mind, but primary care physicians—and cardiologists especially—have not been traditionally trained to recognize and treat psychological issues. The old saying, "If you're a hammer, everything is a nail," describes the tendency for many doctors to look for conditions they've been trained to recognize and are familiar treating. In other words, they're not comfortable delving into potentially uncomfortable territory like personal relationships. "It is odd that we thread catheters, ablate lesions, and give rectal exams but are uncomfortable asking patients about their lives," wrote Joel E. Dimsdale, MD, a psychiatrist at the University of California, San Diego, in an editorial that focused on the link between anxiety and cardiovascular disease.[1]

Thankfully, things are changing, and doctors of all types are realizing that your emotional state needs to be addressed when they ask about and treat your physical symptoms. In fact, most medical training programs now teach trainees to evaluate patients for common psychiatric conditions. On the research level, there has been a growing trend toward examining the link between physical and mental health.

In 1993, researchers at the Montreal Heart Institute in Quebec were one of the first groups to document the connection between depression following a heart attack and mortality rates. They concluded that

"Major depression in patients hospitalized following a [heart attack] is an independent risk factor for mortality at six months. Its impact is at least equivalent to the risk associated with damage caused to the heart muscle or a prior heart attack."[2]

After that research came out, interest in the topic blossomed quickly, so much so that in 2005, researchers out of the Harvard School of Public Health acknowledged that the link between depression and the risk of cardiovascular issues among both the healthy and those with diagnosed cardiac disease was so well established, they wanted to examine lesser known states. Analyzing the "small but emerging literature that has focused on the effects of other negative psychological states on cardiovascular health," they found that five states—hopelessness, pessimism, rumination, anxiety, and anger—have been linked, in varying degrees, to cardiovascular disease or disturbances.[3]

The literature continues to grow. In 2010, doctors out of the University of Pittsburgh reviewed sixty-seven studies that involved at least one hundred women each and focused on *coronary heart disease* (CHD) and negative emotions, stress, social relationships, and positive psychological factors. "Evidence suggests that depression, anxiety disorders, anger suppression, and stress associated with relationships or family responsibilities are associated with elevated coronary heart disease risk among women," they concluded, "[and] supportive social relationships and positive psychological factors may be associated with reduced risk."[4]

Today, there is no question: you are what you feel. I am very cognizant of that when I examine a patient; I ask her about her life, what is going on, what is going wrong, what is giving her joy. I ask my patients to specifically identify what they perceive to be the greatest sources of stress in their lives.

The Physiology Behind Emotional Health

When you feel anything, from happiness to exhaustion, your brain releases chemicals or neurotransmitters, which are essentially like radio waves between cells. One nerve releases the message via neurotransmitter, and, depending on the kind of signal transmitted another nerve receives it (see the chart below). What is happening in the body and mind can affect the quality of the transmission; for example, people who suffer from chronic depression may have a reduced ability to receive the signals. In other words, all of our daily experiences are processed by our nervous system and can actually affect the release and effectiveness of chemicals in our brains.

Common Neurotransmitters

There are over one hundred known neurotransmitters; here are a few of the most common ones that are associated with moods.

NEUROTRANSMITTER	ASSOCIATED WITH
Serotonin	Appetite, sleep, aggression, depression
Norepinephrine	Emotions, learning, dreaming, attentiveness, depression
Dopamine	Motivation, bliss, pleasure, and euphoria; key in positive reinforcement and dependency
GABA (gamma-aminobutyric acid)	Anxiety, panic, pain
Endorphins	Mood elevation, euphoria, natural pain killer; often responsible for "runner's high"
Acetylcholine	Thought, learning, memory, wakefulness, attentiveness, anger, aggression, sexuality

There are three main negative feelings that have been proven to be risk factors for cardiovascular disease: anger, depression, and anxiety. (Stress is another one, but that deserves its own chapter, which starts on page 89.) Balancing them out is a sense of well-being, an overarching emotion that includes happiness, contentment, and positivity.

Anger

"People often think that the type A's—the ones that are always wanting to achieve and can't relax—are the kind to sustain a heart attack," says Kate Traynor, program director of the Cardiovascular Disease Prevention Center at Massachusetts General Hospital, "but that hasn't been my experience. I think people with hostility and cynicism—the really angry people—are the biggest problem." I'm sure you're familiar with the type. They're the ones who count the items in your grocery basket, and if you're one banana over the ten-item limit, they call you on it. They honk (or worse) at you on the highway for the most minor infraction. They complain to managers regularly and never seem to be content. They're so enraged with the world, their anger is almost palpable when you come near them.

Anger does not do your heart any favors. When you become angry, your body reacts as if it's under attack: Your heartbeat picks up as does your blood pressure. Your muscles tense, and stress-related hormones flood your system. You're ready to fight, which creates another problem: that energy your anger has just drummed up has to go somewhere. With no easy outlet save beating up the person with that extra banana—not recommended—anger stays in your body, and eventually your cardiovascular system takes the hit. Anger, hostility, and frustration increase your risk of atrial fibrillation, calcium deposition in the heart arteries, and developing heart symptoms and disease. What's more, if you've already suffered one heart attack, unchecked anger makes you more susceptible to suffering a second one.

Anger doesn't have to be red-faced confrontation for it to influence your body. Looking at 203 women who were hospitalized for an acute cardiac event, Swedish researchers asked the women to fill out an anger questionnaire. Following them for an average of six years, the researchers found that both the women's outward expression *and* their suppression of anger were associated with worsened prognosis of coronary heart disease.[5] In other words, it's not just swearing at your fellow drivers; *wanting to* is equally as dangerous.

If you're a totally healthy person with just a small anger problem, your health still doesn't get a pass. In 2009, English researchers at University College London reviewed forty-four studies that looked at anger in healthy populations and in those people who already have CHD. Examining the various results, they concluded that anger and hostility are associated with coronary heart disease in *both* healthy and CHD populations. In other words, to quote the title of a book that Traynor often recommends to the fuming types, anger kills.[6]

Depression

An international epidemic, depression will be the second most common health problem in the world by the year 2020, according to the World Health Organization.[7] In the States, according to the National Institute of Mental Health, about 7 percent of the population has major depression (defined as a severely depressed mood and activity level that lasts for more than two weeks) at any one time, and the majority of those suffering are women. In fact, women are 70 percent more likely to suffer from depression than men.[8]

This isn't good news for your heart. As mentioned earlier, cardiovascular disease and depression can be a deadly duo. The scientific evidence connecting depression and cardiovascular disease has been so scientifically well established that in 2008 the AHA, in conjunction with the American Psychiatric Association, recommended that all patients diagnosed with coronary heart disease should also be screened for depression.

The exact physiological link between the two diseases is still under investigation—it could be attributed to anything from depression creating more fatty acids in the blood to the connection of more stress and premature atherosclerosis—but some interesting new research out of Emory University in Atlanta uncovered one helpful clue. The researchers focused on *coronary flow reserve*, a measure of the ability of small blood vessels in the heart to relax and dilate as blood flows through them. Looking at sixty-eight pairs of male fraternal twins, where one twin had major depression and the other did not, they found that coronary flow reserve was 14 percent lower in the twin with major depression than in the brothers who were not depressed.[9] Among other things, those small blood vessels help mediate blood pressure in the heart, so when they're not functioning well, neither is your heart. To me, the relationship between compromised coronary flow and depression is a very plausible one.

While the physiological side of things might take a few more years to untangle, it's clear that behavioral factors play a key role in physical health. When you're depressed, it can feel like you're living in quicksand; every action and movement seems to require a Herculean effort. "I get so depressed in the wintertime, it's hard to even get out of bed," says

Susan, a HAPPY Heart participant. As such, people with depression are less likely to take care of themselves. It's easier to forgo exercise, eat poorly, not take your medications, drink too much, and smoke.

Regardless of where exactly the blame for the depression and physical health link lies, the results are clear: your heart is at risk. Researchers are continuing to explore the association. In 2009, doctors at Columbia University Medical Center in New York City found that women who were treated with an antidepressant (a sign of depression) but without any history of heart disease, had an increased risk of sudden cardiac death. (Sudden cardiac death isn't a heart attack, but rather death resulting from an abrupt loss of heart function, which is often caused by coronary heart disease or fatty buildups in the arteries that supply blood to the heart muscle.[10]) In 2010, Swedish researchers looked at women around age thirty who had suffered major depressive episodes, and discovered a premature thickening of their carotid arteries, which is a marker for future cardiovascular events.[11]

In 2010, researchers took data from the British Whitehall II study, which looks at the effect of social and economic factors on the long-term health of civil servants. Looking at the data over a range of five-and-a-half years, they found that people who had only coronary heart disease were 67 percent more likely to die of all causes than their healthy peers, while those who were depressed but had healthy hearts were twice as likely to die than those who were happy and healthy. But the real kicker was that those who had the combination—both depression and heart disease—were almost five times as likely to die as people who had neither affliction. When the researchers adjusted the data for age, sex, and other influential factors, the results were just as troubling. The depression/heart disease combination tripled the risk of death from all causes, and quadrupled a person's chances of dying from a heart attack or stroke.[12]

Not surprisingly, depression that incrementally grows worse also negatively influences your cardiovascular health. In early 2011, a study published in the *Journal of the American College of Cardiology* uncovered a link between worsening depression and poor outcomes in patients with heart failure over the course of one year. Those who had the greatest increase in depression had more than twice the risk of cardiovascular-related hospitalization or death, compared to those patients whose depression had plateaued or stabilized.[13]

What makes all these facts and studies so much more disturbing is that after you hear you have heart disease or suffer a heart attack, you're much more prone to depression. Studies vary, but it appears that somewhere between one-third to one-half of patients experience depression in the first year following heart surgery. In addition, researchers in 2009 looked at the relationship between a new diagnosis of depression after a diagnosis of coronary artery disease in over 13,700 patients. Ten percent of the study group was diagnosed with depression. Subsequently, 16.4 percent of the depressed individuals were diagnosed with heart failure, compared to only 3.6 percent of those without depression.[14]

As a cancer survivor, I completely understand that response: cancer and heart problems aren't like pneumonia or appendicitis, which can be treated relatively quickly or forgotten. They—or at least the threat of them—never go away. When I first give a patient in my office the news that her heart isn't healthy, I can usually see in her eyes that she recognizes that she has crossed the threshold from health to unhealth. Even if she's a fit, healthy person, a diagnosis of cardiac disease automatically forces her to cross the bridge from being a healthy person to a patient. She will be a patient for the rest of her life, and that news is not easy to stomach, especially if she's a young person who still has her whole life in front of her.

A Depression Screen

The Patient Health Questionnaire is a simple nine-question test that is often administered by physicians. I've included it here because it's a basic test that can indicate if you're suffering from depression.

Over the last two weeks, how often have you been bothered by any of the following problems?

	QUESTION	NOT AT ALL	SEVERAL DAYS	MORE THAN HALF THE DAYS	NEARLY EVERY DAY
1	Little interest or pleasure in doing things	0	1	2	3
2	Feeling down, depressed, or hopeless	0	1	2	3
3	Trouble falling asleep, staying asleep, or sleeping too much	0	1	2	3
4	Feeling tired or having little energy	0	1	2	3
5	Poor appetite or overeating	0	1	2	3
6	Feeling bad about yourself, that you are a failure, or that you have let yourself or your family down	0	1	2	3
7	Trouble concentrating on things such as reading the newspaper or watching television	0	1	2	3
8	Moving or speaking so slowly that other people could have noticed or being so fidgety or restless that you have been moving around a lot more than usual	0	1	2	3
9	Thinking that you would be better off dead or that you want to hurt yourself in some way	0	1	2	3

Score Yourself: If you answered question 1 or 2 as either "more than half the days" or "nearly every day," continue. If you answered "not at all" or "several days," you can stop scoring.

If you answered question 9 with anything other than "not at all," you need to speak to your primary care physician about whether counseling, antidepressant medication, and/or psychiatric care are warranted as soon as possible.

- Add up the numbers in the "several days" column.

  Total: _____

- Add up the numbers in the "more than half the days" column and multiply by 2.

  Total: _____

- Add up the numbers in the "nearly every day" column and multiply by 3.

  Total: _____

- Add up your three totals.

  Total: _____

If you scored more than 10, you should be aware that you have some mild symptoms of possible depression, and the higher your score, the potentially worse your situation is; speak to your physician about this if things worsen. To ease the symptoms, do your best to take the *Smart at Heart* approach to life with diet, exercise, and stress management.

The good news is that treatments for depression have come a long way over the past few decades. The first generation of antidepressants had the potential for severe cardiac side effects, including sudden death. They virtually scared cardiologists to death; we thought that it was better to live with depression than die trying to fight it. Fast-forward to the fourth generation of antidepressants, which are currently on the market and have been improved greatly; they are now safe for most individuals. Still, the perceived threat from earlier medications hangs like smoke in the air. I routinely see cardiac patients who are sent by their primary care physicians for a consultation so they can be cleared to take an antidepressant.

Anxiety

It's not as well researched or as frequently discussed as anger and depression, but anxiety is quickly becoming another emotion that can have a negative effect on your cardiac health. In June 2010, the *Journal of the American College of Cardiology* looked at the issue in depth. In an editorial, Joel E. Dimsdale, MD, calls anxiety "toxic to the cardiovascular system," which is an audacious and scary statement, considering he then notes that anxiety disorders are as prevalent as hypertension, and its impact on the body's overall functioning is roughly akin to that of lower back pain or leg ulcers. When anxiety coexists with depression, the corresponding impact on quality of life "is even worse," he observes, "along the lines of the impact of chronic obstructive pulmonary disease."[15]

Anxiety is similar to anger; both bring on the same flood of stress-related hormones and accompanying tenseness and virtual clinching of the cardiac system. But anxiety is worse, as it can also be associated with panic attacks, that out-of-control sensation that brings on a rapid heartbeat, sweating, and even breathlessness. (Of course, these symptoms can also be associated with a medical condition, so if they last more than a few minutes you should seek medical attention.)

The severe impact anxiety has on the cardiovascular system has been of scientific interest lately. In a study published in 2010, researchers in the Netherlands merged data from twenty studies that included approximately 250,000 people from around the world. Adjusting for all the factors like age, sex, and previous health conditions that could influence the data, they concluded that anxious people had around a 25 percent greater risk of heart disease and an almost 50 percent higher risk of cardiac death over a mean follow-up period of 11.2 years.[16]

In a study published in 2008, doctors looked at the relationship between anxiety and heart attacks in 735 American middle-aged or elderly men who were in good cardiovascular health in 1986. They asked the men to fill out four different scales to gauge their anxiety and found that those whose anxiety scores put them in the top 15 percent on one scale or on a combined scale of all four, were 30 to 40 percent more likely to have a heart attack than those who were less anxious.[17]

When to Seek Help

Despite what you may think, counseling is not the twenty-first-century equivalent of a scarlet A. "Therapy is a health prescription," says Susan Lane, RN, MSN, MBA, a health educator with HAPPY Heart. "I often tell people who are wary of it to think of it this way: If you were running a company, you would bring in advisers, lawyers, accountants, and other people to maximize your success. Now think of your body as a company: wouldn't you want to employ people to get your body in the best place possible?"

When do you know it might be time to talk to a professional? If you feel depressed, anxious, lonely, or angry more often than not, or when you're unable to function the way you normally do, a therapist can certainly help. An objective opinion can also be beneficial when you're going through relationship problems, have issues with your career, feel stuck in life, or are experiencing a major life transition (a death of a parent, a divorce, a birth, an isolating move). Another easy way to answer that question is if something in your life has you debating about speaking to a helpful third party, it's worth one session.

Counselors, therapists, psychiatrists, and psychologists are trained not only to provide a safe, professional environment where you can have a confidential discussion about the parts of your life that need work, but also to help you decide whether the counseling process is all you need or whether antianxiety or antidepressant medications may be needed.

How do you find a mental health professional? Many employers offer employee assistance programs that can provide referrals; your doctor may also have some. A trusted friend or family member is also a good person to ask. If you have health insurance, they will have a list of professionals in your area. If you don't, check at a public health clinic or center where session cost may be based on income.

Well-Being

So it's painfully clear how catastrophic the negative emotions can be on the physical body, but what about the positive emotions? The science of happiness has become increasingly more substantial and convincing and points to a robust link between happiness and health. In early 2011, Ed Diener, PhD, a pioneer in the well-being field and professor emeritus of psychology at the University of Illinois, led a review of more than 160 studies that involve human and animal subjects and some aspect of health and subjective well-being (life satisfaction, absence of negative emotions, optimism, and positive emotions). It was released in *Applied Psychology: Health and Well-Being*. "The general conclusion from each type of study is that your subjective well-being—that is, feeling positive about your life, not stressed, not depressed—contributes to both longevity and better health among healthy populations," Diener said.[18] The 160 studies spanned subjects from nuns to monkeys to university students. "I was almost shocked and certainly surprised to see the consistency of data," Diener told *Science Daily*. "All of these different kinds of studies point to the same conclusion: that health and then longevity in turn are influenced by our mood states." He then added that "happiness is no magic bullet, but the evidence is clear and compelling that it changes your odds of getting disease or dying young."[19]

One of the most often-cited studies regarding emotions and physical health is one headed up by Sheldon Cohen, a psychology professor at Carnegie Mellon University in Pittsburgh, Pennsylvania. Cohen and his colleagues interviewed volunteers over several weeks to assess their moods and emotional styles and then infected them with either a rhinovirus or influenza virus. They were then quarantined and examined. The researchers found the people who were happy, lively, and calm—or otherwise exhibited positive emotions—were less likely to become ill than those who reported few of those emotions. "We need to take more seriously the possibility that positive emotional style is a major player in disease risk," Cohen commented.[20]

Following in the wake of Cohen's study, a multitude of studies have reinforced the message that the happier you are, the better your health likely is. Researchers in the United Kingdom and Texas tracked

823 people aged fifty-five years or older who had suffered a stroke to examine the link between positive attitude and improved recovery after a devastating health crisis. Checking in with patients three months after the stroke, those who had more positive emotions were found to have a higher overall functional status as well as improved mental and physical states, compared to those with glass-half-empty outlooks.[21] Similarly, nearly ten thousand Australians were asked about their level of contentment with simple questions ("During the past four weeks, have you been a happy person?" "All things considered, how satisfied are you with your life?"). Those who answered that they were happy or satisfied also reported that they had excellent, very good, or good health and no limiting health conditions.[22]

One aspect of good health was measured in more medical terms in a study that examined the correlation between psychological well-being and high blood pressure in sixteen European countries. Using two simple questions—"Would you say that you have had problems of high blood pressure?" and "Would you say that you are very satisfied, fairly satisfied, not very satisfied, or not at all satisfied with the life you lead?"—the researchers used the results to conclude that the "happier" countries report less hypertension. (Sweden and Denmark topped the list of happiness and low blood pressure, while Germany and Portugal brought up the rear.) The correlation was so strong, the authors suggest that blood pressure readings might form an element in a national well-being index.[23]

As I was finishing this chapter, we got some new data from the HAPPY heart study: after one year in the study, the women demonstrated a significant decrease in their levels of stress, depression, and anxiety, compared to when they entered the program. That's good news on many levels.

Three Easy First Steps Across the Emotional Health Bridge

1. **Don't relive the drama.** You may have had a drag-it-out fight with your daughter, you may have been rear-ended at a stoplight, and you may have continual chaos at your job. Obviously, it's best to rectify these situations at the source, but until you do that, do your best not to retell the stories over and over again. "I felt like the negative talk manifested itself," says Joyce, a member of HAPPY Heart who was in a serious car accident and had to recount her story to plenty of doctors and lawyers after the accident. "When you're always talking about what is hurting you, it becomes a negative force. I couldn't stop dwelling on it." The negative force isn't just a mental handicap; as you relive events that cause anger or anxiety, your body reacts negatively as well.

2. **Try not to create drama.** When a patient tells me that the greatest sources of stress in her lives are others and how they treat her, I remind her that others cannot make her feel bad without her permission. Or, as health coach Donna Slicis says, "You can't change a situation or a person, but you can change how you react to it." With every interaction you are in, you have a choice: you can become way too invested and interpret everything in a personal manner or you can try to be more objective and less emotional about it.

3. **Practice random acts of kindness.** British researchers confirmed the merits of the popular bumper sticker when they grouped adults, ages eighteen to sixty, into three categories: for ten days, one group would perform an act of kindness to a stranger, one group would do something novel,

and one group would not change their daily routine. After ten days, the groups that either reached out to strangers or did something new and different reported an increase in life satisfaction, while the other group did not.[24] Pay somebody's toll behind you, pound some nails for Habitat for Humanity, pick fresh lilacs for a friend, or otherwise do something new and/or kind, and your perspective will perk up accordingly.

chapter four

The Stress Management Bridge

"Oh, do I know about stress," says Kara, a fifty-seven-year-old woman who is definitely not a drama queen. Name a typical stress, and Kara had it—in spades. An ailing parent? Yes. Her ninety-one-year-old mother, who was dying from breast cancer, among other things, came to live with Kara for eight months before she passed away. "That sucked the life out of me," she says. Financial worries? Check. When her mother moved in, Kara was going to school to get a degree in accounting. "But I had to drop out to care for my mom," she says. "It was too hard to do everything." Plus her three boys, all in their early twenties, were still in school—college, in fact. "We took out loans for their educations," she says. "It's so expensive, it's crazy. The numbers just sit on my brain, burdening it." Relationship strife? Been there. Her ex-husband was an abusive alcoholic. "I left him in 1997," she says, "the day I started a program in domestic violence." During her time with him, and afterward, as she tried to put herself back together, "I just lost myself," she admits. "I started to put on weight and fell into the same pattern as my mother, who went to her grave overweight. I fell into a rut and couldn't get out." Little social support? Positive. "Because of my weight, I rarely interacted with people outside of my family," says Kara. "I spent my days playing solitaire on the computer." Other significant life changes? Unfortunately, yes. Her older brother passed away recently too. "I ate three birthday cakes when he died," she remembers, "and I went out to eat every single day. Who wants to cook then anyway?"

At 241 pounds, Kara, whose father died of a heart attack when she was seven, couldn't really afford to eat those birthday cakes. Fortunately, between the times her mother and brother died, she joined the HAPPY Heart program. "I'd never taken care of my health before," she says. "I just hoped for the best." That strategy, combined with the crazy stress in her life, obviously wasn't very successful. Finally ready to lose weight, Kara asked her primary care physician for some advice, and she gave her a referral to a nutritionist, who mentioned the program. "My mom was gone, my kids are grown, it's time to take care of me," she said. "Enough is enough." So willing to get started, to do something to lighten her load, change something in the hopes that it might spark something else, she immediately said, "I'll do it."

For decades, Kara lived with chronic stress. Her metaphorical load was as heavy as her body became, and her body undeniably paid the price. Our bodies can thrive under small amounts of stress, but they're not built to handle chronic stress.

This Is Your Body on Stress

Stress, in its simplest sense, is the body's normal response to change. That change can be short-term (a good thing) or chronic, lingering on for weeks, months, and years (a not-so-good thing). When you feel stressed, your body gets ready to either fight or flee; our bodies are wired the same way our ancestors were. When they entered a stressful situation—a predator, a lack of food, a natural disaster—they either had to defend themselves or get the heck out of there. Our bodies don't know the difference between a saber-toothed tiger and a job interview, so they react in the same agitated way they would've a thousand years ago, by entering into fight-or-flight mode. Whether you feel stressed because of a nearby car that cuts you off or the anticipation of going home to your moody teenage daughter, your chain reaction begins and the adrenal glands above the kidneys release the hormones nor-epinephrine, epinephrine (or adrenalin), and cortisol. As they hit your bloodstream, your blood pressure and heart rate rise, the glucose levels in your blood elevate so you can easily access energy, your muscles tense, your breathing becomes faster, and your senses become sharper. With those parts of your body getting ready to rumble, other less necessary parts, like your digestive, reproductive, and immune systems, slow or shut down. Once the threat has passed, the body calms down; stress hormones return to normal, as do all the body's systems.

Not all stress is bad; in fact, stress can give us a sense of purpose and make us feel alive and excited. A first date, especially if it goes well, is a great example. Even short-term episodes of unfavorable stress (a job interview that doesn't go well, traffic moving at a glacial pace) aren't typically bad for your health. If the stress has a starting point (when a first date or interview starts, when you get on the highway) and ending point (when the date or interview ends, when you eventually exit the highway) and you don't dwell on it for hours after, your physical health is unscathed.

Chronic stress, however, is a different story. Chronic stress is the inescapable, suffocating kind, like Kara experienced, the kind that doesn't naturally work itself out or feel less burdensome with time. It could be stress from a troubling marriage, a relationship with an ailing family member, or a job situation that never feels easy or enjoyable. With the other types of stress, your body recovers and can go back to its relaxed, normal state. With chronic stress, because the stress never disappears, your body is continually ready to fight; your fists might not be clenched all day long, but it certainly feels like they are.

I think stress levels are as important as blood pressure readings and cholesterol numbers. According to the American Psychological Association (APA), 75 to 90 percent of all physician office visits are for stress-related ailments and complaints. That statistic makes sense, given that the APA notes that 43 percent of all adults suffer adverse health effects from stress.[1] Compared to those who consider themselves in excellent or very good health, people who rate their health as fair or poor are more likely to experience stress-related symptoms like anger, exhaustion, little motivation or energy, poor sleep, and overeating.[2] Women, in particular, are more prone to the ill effects of stress; the APA notes that females are more likely than males to experience headaches, stomach-related issues, or sadness when they feel stressed. Married women seem to carry the most stress, with one in three married women having high levels of stress, compared to one in five single women.[3]

Before you read any further, please remember that you can't eliminate stress in your life. What stresses you can change through your life—my younger patients tend to worry about finances, careers, and caring for their children and parents, while my older ones worry about their health and independence—but stress itself can't. Unlike other bridges—like nutrition, exercise, and communication where you can proactively make positive changes and leave negative habits behind (for example, bypassing the chocolate chip cookies, walking daily, and choosing not to interact with negative people), you can't choose to live in a stress-free world. (Well, you could, but that means no families, no pets, no interaction with the world, no driving, no working . . . and what fun is that?) What's more, life experiences can make you more prone to stress; for instance, if you were abused as a child, research has shown that you might be more vulnerable to reacting poorly to other stressful events.

What you can do, however, is decide that you will downsize the sources of chronic stress and develop coping mechanisms that don't allow stress to "metastasize" in your body. Before I suggest ways to do that, I want to cover the symptoms of stress, how to gauge your stress level, and the physical effects stress has on the body.

Test Your Stress

While there are a variety of stress questionnaires out there, we use this Perceived Stress Scale in HAPPY Heart; I like it because it is well validated, simple, and comes in English and Spanish versions.

Go through and answer the questions using the following scale:

0 = Never
1 = Almost never
2 = Sometimes
3 = Fairly often
4 = Very often

1. In the last month, how often have you been upset because of something that happened unexpectedly?

2. In the last month, how often have you felt that you were unable to control the important things in your life?

3. In the last month, how often have you felt nervous and "stressed"?

4. In the last month, how often have you dealt successfully with irritating life hassles?

5. In the last month, how often have you felt that you were effectively coping with important changes that were occurring in your life?

6. In the last month, how often have you felt confident about your ability to handle your personal problems?

7. In the last month, how often have you felt that things were going your way?

8. In the last month, how often have you found that you could not cope with all the things that you had to do?

9. In the last month, how often have you been able to control irritations in your life?

10. In the last month, how often have you felt that you were on top of things?

11. In the last month, how often have you been angered because of things that were outside of your control?

12. In the last month, how often have you found yourself thinking about things that you have to accomplish?

13. In the last month, how often have you been able to control the way you spend your time?

14. In the last month, how often have you felt difficulties were piling up so high that you could not overcome them?

Add up your score:

- For questions 1, 2, 3, 8, 11, 12, and 14, use the number you wrote down.

- For questions 4, 5, 6, 7, 9, 10, and 13, use this scale to convert your responses:

  4 = 0, 3 = 1, 2 = 2, 1 = 3, 0 = 4.

In the initial study that was published in 1983, the average score for the 299 women polled was 25.6. Cohen has since done samples of a similar, 10-question stress test in 1983, 2006, and 2009. His results conclude that "the distributions of stress remained virtually identical across the three surveys (26 years). In all cases women reported greater stress than men; stress decreased with increasing age, education, and income; and minorities tended to report more stress than whites. The unemployed reported more stress than the employed in 1983 and 2006 but not in 2009 [year of economic recession] and the retired reported the lowest level of stress across employment categories in all three surveys."[4] If you find yourself with a higher score, it is certainly concerning and an indication of overwhelming stress. Discuss your situation with your doctor.

The PSS scale is reprinted with permission of the American Sociological Association, from S. Cohen, T. Kamarck, and R. Mermelstein, "A Global Measure of Perceived Stress," *Journal of Health and Social Behavior* 24 (1983): 386-396.

Symptoms of Stress

Stress can appear in many forms in your body, mind, and day-to-day life. Here's a list of the most common symptoms of stress. If you have more than one of these symptoms on a regular basis, there is a good chance there is too much stress in your life. In other words, it's time to make some changes before stress wreaks havoc with your health.

PHYSICAL	PSYCHOLOGICAL	BEHAVIORAL
Insomnia	Sadness/depression	Teeth grinding
Headaches	Irritability	Frequent crying
Loss of sex drive	Anger	Rapid speaking
Weight loss or gain	Frustration	Fast-paced walking
Neck or back pain	Anxiety	Alcohol or drug abuse
GI distress	Difficulty concentrating	Excessive smoking
Fainting/feeling light-headed or dizzy	Restlessness	Less likely to take medications as prescribed
Fatigue		Binge eating or eating unhealthy foods
Palpitations or shortness of breath*		
Chest pressure*		

*Both of these symptoms can have other causes, so please get them checked out by a doctor.

This Is Your Body on Chronic Stress

What happens when stress becomes the rule in your life and not the exception—when you eat most meals over a keyboard or a steering wheel because you always have something to do or somewhere to be, when your nighttime reading material is your work for the next day, when your relationships cause you more worry than happiness? Here's a hint: it's not pretty.

Here's a run-down of what unchecked stress can do to your body.

Chronic Stress Puts You at Increased Risk for Heart Disease

Physically, it causes your heart rate and blood pressure to stay consistently elevated. In addition, the stress hormones cause your blood vessels to constrict so your heart has to work harder to push blood through smaller-than-usual channels. The hormones secreted with it increase the stickiness of blood cells, making them more likely to clot, which in turn, increases the risk of heart attack and stroke.

Chronic Stress Also Speeds Up the Process of Atherosclerosis

Platelets in the blood, mobilized by stress hormones, go to the site of damaged arteries to heal them. LDL cholesterol is also naturally drawn to the arteries; the combination of the two causes the arterial walls to thicken, which, in turn, can result in premature atherosclerosis.

Recent studies bear this out. Looking at the relationship between job stress and strain, job insecurity, and cardiovascular disease in 17,415 women, researchers in Boston found that women who reported high job strain were 40 percent more likely to experience a cardiovascular disease–related event than those who reported low job strain. Those with high job insecurity didn't have their risk of cardiovascular disease go up, but they were more likely to smoke, be sedentary, have a high BMI, and be at risk for diabetes, high blood pressure, and high cholesterol.[5] In other words, chronic stress related to fighting a stressor, like job strain, or just giving up and accepting the status quo, like living with job insecurity, have detrimental health effects.

Another study looked at the effect of work and marital stress and the incidence of coronary heart disease for 292 women in Sweden. The researchers found that those who were either married or living with a partner were nearly three times more likely to have another coronary event.[6] Interestingly, work stress didn't predict another coronary event but the fact that in Sweden, an egalitarian society where women are given a year off after giving birth and work doesn't dominate as it does in the United States, job stressors have less of a negative impact on health and are worth considering. I think if the same study were conducted in the States, both sources of stress—work and relationship—would be significant.

Chronic Stress Speeds Effects of Aging

Although this relationship was long suspected, it was confirmed less than a decade ago, in 2004, when scientists at the University of California at San Francisco looked at thirty-nine women, ages twenty to fifty, who were caring for a child with a serious chronic illness (like autism or cerebral palsy) and were therefore under extreme stress. The scientists looked at *telomeres*, structures in cells that are positioned on the end of chromosomes and get shorter with every division of a cell. When a cell has no more telomeres, it can't divide, it dies, and the corresponding part of the body—skin, muscles, organs, eyesight, brain function—ages. They also looked at *telomerase*, an enzyme that boosts the telomere's life span. Compared to women who had healthy kids, the thirty-nine had shorter telomeres and less telomerase; the longer a woman had been caring for her child, the more drastic her telomere situation was. In addition, they found that the women with the highest levels of perceived stress had the telomeres of a person ten years older than them, confirming the mind-body connection.[7]

Chronic Stress Compromises Your Immune System

Under stress, wounds are slower to heal and the body is more susceptible to colds and flu. A handful of studies have shown that stress reduces the body's ability to produce antibodies in response to a vaccine (hepatitis B in younger people, pneumococcal vaccines in the elderly), which makes the body more vulnerable to infections.[8]

Chronic Stress Causes Your Inflammation Markers to Rise

In turn, your risk for coronary artery disease, atherosclerosis, high blood pressure, insulin resistance, kidney disease, asthma, allergies, rheumatoid arthritis, and lupus all increase. A landmark study in 2003 followed caregivers who tended to a spouse or loved one with dementia for six years. The caregivers' levels of *Interleukin-6* (IL-6)—a marker of inflammation that is associated with cardiovascular disease, osteoporosis, arthritis, type 2 diabetes, certain cancers, and periodontal disease, among others—were four times higher than that of controls who had the same age, sex, health, and socioeconomic status. What's more troubling is that the difference in IL-6 levels remained for several years after the caregiving stopped.[9]

Chronic Stress Increases Your Risk of Osteoporosis

Cortisol, one of the major stress hormones, can pull calcium from your bones, which puts you at risk for developing osteoporosis. In 2009, researchers in Italy examined the relationship between stress hormones and low bone density in 481 people. Looking at the x-rays of the hip bone and the lumbar spine, they found that those people with high cortisol levels had significantly lower bone density and, as such, were at higher risk for fractures.[10]

Chronic Stress Could Increase Your Risk for Cancer

A 2008 study out of Israel had some compelling, albeit troubling, results about the link between stress and cancer. Comparing 255 women under age forty-five who had been diagnosed with breast cancer with 367 of their healthy counterparts, the researchers asked both groups how many severe life changes—for instance, loss of a parent, spouse or close relative, loss of a job, an economic crisis, separation or divorce—they experienced. Looking at the data, the researchers found the risk of breast cancer increased by 62 percent in women who had undergone more than one significant life change.[11]

Chronic Stress Makes You More Likely to Gain Weight

Left unchecked, stress can pile on the pounds. Not only does feeling stressed make you more likely to crave sugar and fat, the stress hormones raise the glucose levels in your blood. When you don't burn up that glucose to fight or flee, it is prone to settle into your midsection, which is the least ideal place, from a health perspective, for it to be stored. Researchers at Wake Forest University School of Medicine in Winston-Salem, North Carolina, confirmed this in 2009, when they carried out an experiment with female primates. All were fed a Western-style diet and then were housed in groups so they would naturally establish a social hierarchy, from dominant to subordinate.

The monkeys on the lowest rungs of the social ladder, who were often the target of aggression and weren't included in group grooming sessions, developed more fat in their abdomen (viscera fat).[12] That kind of fat is tied to coronary artery atherosclerosis, as well as diabetes, heart disease, and metabolic syndrome.

Research on humans also points to a strong connection between stress and weight gain. Using data from the 1,355 men and women across the United States who participated in the nine-year, comprehensive Midlife in the United States (MIDUS) study, researchers at Harvard in 2009 looked at the correlation between stress and weight gain. They found a particularly noticeable relationship with men and women who had high baseline body mass indexes (a BMI of about 27.5 for men and 26 for women). Women who were overweight were more likely to gain weight if they felt stress from job-related demands, perceived constraints in life, strain in family relations, and difficulty paying bills.[13]

Chronic Stress Makes You More Susceptible to Depression and Anxiety

Like a knotted-up ball of yarn, it's hard to know where stress ends and serious conditions like depression and anxiety begin. Plenty of studies have established a link between stress, depression, and anxiety; in early 2011, researchers performed a literature review of studies that involved cardiovascular disease in women, anxiety, and depression.

They concluded that family stress was increased in the women with increased levels of depression and anxiety. Improved quality of life, on the other hand, was linked to lower levels of depression, anxiety, and angina.[14]

The Bridge to Stress Management

I love the sentiment of a popular Chinese proverb: in the times of crisis, we are allowed the greatest opportunities for change. Chronic stress is definitely a time of crisis, and if you can take a step back and a deep breath, you can drastically change how you react to and process stress. Here are some ideas for you to reduce your stress levels.

Forget Perfection

Easier said than done, I realize, if you're the type who has ambitious standards that you can never seem to meet. Not to knock you down, but chances are, you'll never be satisfied. When you do meet one standard, instead of reveling in your success, you're likely already looking forward to your next challenge. One of my favorite phrases is "Better is the enemy of good." Most of the time, good is good enough. I have spent much of my life around people who seek perfection and I'll be honest: I found most of those folks weren't very happy.

Be Grateful for the Stress

Realize that the things that can bring you the most joy and satisfaction—your family, your house, your job—can also be the biggest sources of stress. When your kid is up all night with a fever, your dishwasher breaks, or a new set of responsibilities is handed to you at work, you can, of course, feel stressed. Or you can also mentally zoom out, and remember that this will pass and, although it sounds corny, you can consider yourself lucky to have such problems.

The Need for Sleep

As a rule, the women I see in my practice undervalue sleep. There's so much to be done and only so many hours in the day; left to choose between productivity and rest, most people opt for the former, despite the fact that your ability to efficiently finish any task goes down exponentially with lack of sleep.

When you opt for late-night reruns or writing emails over shut-eye, your body and mind suffer. A lack of sleep has been scientifically linked to depression, changes in memory, a weakened immune system, and a decreased ability to concentrate. One study found that women who slept eight hours a night had lower levels of the inflammatory marker IL-6, which may be linked to heart disease; a direct connection has not been established yet. Women who slept for seven hours had higher levels, and women who clocked in at less than five hours nightly had the highest levels.[15]

Physically, too little sleep also alters how your body regulates your appetite. In 2010, researchers at the University of Chicago did a study that followed ten overweight people who were all on a calorie-restricted diet. For two weeks, five were told to sleep eight-and-half hours a night, and five were told to sleep five-and-a-half hours. While both groups lost weight, the group that got less sleep lost muscle weight instead of fat. More importantly, within two weeks, there were noticeable differences in the sleep-deprived group's levels of the hormones *ghrelin* and *leptin*; ghrelin stimulates the appetite, while leptin is responsible for feeling satisfied. With their hormones out of balance, the tired group was consistently more hungry.[16]

The cycle can be vicious. "You don't sleep, so you gain weight, which makes you have sleep apnea, which causes what little sleep you do get to become even worse, so more stress hormones flood your system, making you insulin resistant," says Donna Slicis. "You're irritable and depressed. You go to the doctor, and because you're depressed, she puts you on an antidepressant, which further interferes with your sleeping."

The opposite is also true: a great night's sleep can unkink many other issues in your life. One HAPPY Heart participant noticed a significant decrease in her anxiety levels when she started to practice sleep hygiene, while another, on a healthier diet and five-day-a-week exercise routine, upped her sleeping to eight hours a night and feels the difference every morning.

Here are some ideas to maximize your sleep:

- If you're consistently waking up after a full night's rest but feel exhausted, have your doctor check you for sleep apnea, a condition where your airway is blocked and your breathing is compromised. "If you're not breathing, you're not sleeping," says Slicis. Attributes of those at risk for sleep apnea include being male, over age forty, and overweight, but it can happen to anybody, and it's serious: it increases the risk of high blood pressure, heart attack, stroke, obesity, and diabetes.

- Get exercise. Yet another benefit of moving your body: it makes it easier to relax and sleep well. Just don't exercise more than four hours before your bedtime or you may feel too jazzed to sleep.

- If you can't shut off your mind to go to sleep, make a worry box. Write down all your worries on small pieces of paper prior to bed, worry about them for a few moments, and then put them in the box. Then don't worry about them anymore since you can't solve anything in your sleep—and you can't solve anything during the day if you're not well rested.

- Realize you sleep in ninety-minute cycles and that you may wake up in between those cycles. In other words, don't freak out because you're awake. "Just reframe your waking," says

Susan Lane. "Think, 'I just finished a cycle. I'll roll over and go back to sleep.'"

- Keep your bedroom screen-free. No computers, no gadgets, no televisions. Use your bed just for sleeping and sex. Some experts recommend that people who have sleep problems shouldn't even read in bed.

- Don't drink caffeine after 2 p.m. and no alcohol after dinner. Both interfere with the body's natural ability to have a productive night's sleep. In addition, try to limit your sugar intake in the afternoon and evening as well.

- Two hours before bedtime, start to turn off any overhead lights and lower other lights around your house. Do something quiet, like reading a book, talking with a friend on the phone, or watching television. An hour before, start your bedtime ritual: wash your face, brush your teeth, and otherwise signal to your body and mind that you're winding down. "So many people wait until the second before they get into bed to start to relax, and then they wonder why they can't sleep," says Lane.

- Try to stay on a set schedule. Get up around the same time every morning, and go to bed around the same time every evening. If your current schedule doesn't allow for the seven to eight hours of sleep you ideally need—say, you have to get up by 7 a.m. for work, but you usually don't go to bed until 1 a.m.—adjust your bedtime by fifteen-minute increments to gradually ease your body into an earlier bedtime.

- If you haven't fallen asleep after twenty or so minutes, get up and do something "really boring," says Lane. "Wash the dishes or read a dull book." Keep the lights low so you don't send the wrong signal to your inner clock.

- Detoxify your diet. Several years ago I followed a strictly macrobiotic diet for three months. I had read a great deal about the health benefits of not eating processed foods. Given my busy schedule and that I was also cooking for four children, a strictly macrobiotic diet did not end up being practical for me, but I did see a dramatic improvement in my sleep habits after cleaning up my diet. Try to eliminate as many processed foods as possible and see if it leads to improved sleep.

Breathe Deeply

When I returned to performing heart catheterizations after moving to Canada and giving birth to my third child, I was very anxious. I was running a household with three small kids, my husband was working eighty hours a week, I had few friends or social support, and I was working on people's hearts in an entirely new environment. I knew I had the training and expertise, but I still wanted to be at the top of my game. During this time, I visited a stress management person at the hospital where I was working, and she gave me a simple handbook about deep, rhythmic breathing. We lived close enough to the hospital that I could walk there, and on my walk, I would center myself with deep, deliberate breathing. I will discuss the techniques of incorporating breathing into your efforts at relaxation in the discussion of the relaxation response (see opposite). Afterward, I felt ready to work and, without fear, was able to focus on the tasks I was trained to do.

Health educator Susan Lane likes to talk about being in the "float," which is in direct contrast to fight or flight. "Within three deep breaths, the body is signaling the mind to go to a float place: to relax and calm down," she says, adding that it's important to practice deep breathing at least five times a day: try it at regular times like before you eat, after you eat, when you go to bed, when you wake up. "Eventually, your body will get in the habit," she says, "and go there with little thought from you."

The Relaxation Response

A pioneer in the field of mind-body medicine, Dr. Herbert Benson opened the Benson-Henry Mind/Body Medical Institute at Massachusetts General Hospital in Boston. When the Wellness Center opened in Revere, he came to the celebration and led us through the Relaxation Response he created, a simple, proven way to get your body and mind centered and calm.

1. Sit quietly in a comfortable position. No need to sit cross-legged, but avoid lying down so you don't fall asleep.

2. Close your eyes.

3. Deeply relax all your muscles, beginning at your feet and progressing up to your face. Keep them relaxed.

4. Breathe through your nose. Become aware of your breathing. As you breathe out, say the word *one*—or any other one-syllable, neutral word that doesn't summon up particular thoughts from you—silently to yourself. With each inhale and exhale, repeat the word. Breathe easily and naturally.

5. Continue for ten to twenty minutes. You may open your eyes to check the time, but do not use an alarm. When you finish, sit quietly for several minutes, first with your eyes closed, then with your eyes open. Do not stand up for a few minutes.

6. During the session, do not worry about whether you are successful in achieving a deep level of relaxation. Instead,

maintain a passive attitude and permit relaxation to occur at its own pace. When—not if—distracting thoughts occur, try to ignore them by not dwelling upon them. Just focus on your breath and word.

Practice the technique once or twice daily, but not within two hours of finishing any meal, since the digestive processes seem to interfere with the effectiveness of the Relaxation Response.[17]

Take to the Sidewalks

One of the cheapest and most effective ways to minimize stress is to go for a brisk walk. Walking gets your heart pumping and your muscles moving, and it leads to deeper, faster breathing. Often a head-clearing activity, it allows for a break from the moment-to-moment stress that can dominate our lives. Getting out of our chairs and moving gives us the subconscious message that we are working to improve our health and the simple knowledge that we are making a good choice is beneficial to our overall demeanor.

When you want to sweat the stress out, a surprising study shows that a walk or similar low-intensity exercise might be the way to go. Looking at the relationship between cortisol levels and exercise intensity, researchers at the University of North Carolina at Chapel Hill found that higher-intensity exercise (80 percent of your maximum heart rate—or, in other words, sprinting, jumping rope, riding a bike very fast) provokes an increase in cortisol levels, while lower-intensity (40 percent of max heart rate, or a brisk walk or moderate swim) does not.[18] This should not dissuade you from participating in brisk aerobic exercise. Rather, it just makes the point that if you are going to exercise, you should do it regularly so that your body adapts to the changes associated with exercise.

Try Yoga

A practice that can be done at any fitness and experience level, yoga is renowned for its calming, centering effects—even on kids. A 2010 study documented the effects of yoga on 122 Israeli schoolchildren, age eight to twelve years, and their six teachers, after the Second Lebanon War. In an effort to reduce tension in the kids who lived in the area under bombardment, the children did thirteen yoga sessions over four months. "The teachers reported many statistically significant improvements in the children's concentration, mood, and ability to function under pressure," the researchers concluded.[19] While this study was done with schoolchildren, a captive audience with which it is easy to follow up, similar results would be expected in adults.

Look for Some Job Control

One of the biggest reasons jobs can feel so stressful is that you're often not the one in control: a supervisor or spreadsheet or something else dictates what you have to get done that day. A recent study showed, for the first time, that maintaining some control over your job can make a difference in stress levels. Researchers had seventy-seven people "work" at a simulated computer workplace for more than two hours and then altered their job demands and control levels. The results showed that even if a job was demanding, if a person felt a high level of control, she didn't show the same levels of stress that somebody who felt a low level of control did.[20] Although you can't kick your boss out of the office, consider ways you might be able to have more autonomy in the workplace; for example, can you head up a project that interests you?

Get a Massage or Acupuncture

You don't need to spend money on an hour-long session at a spa; a calming back rub from a spouse or a simple chair massage at the mall can do wonders for your stress levels. Researchers at Dillard University in New Orleans studied the effects of a chair massage, as well as deep breathing, on African-American women's levels of blood pressure, stress, and anxiety. All three markers decreased in response to receiving massage.[21]

Acupuncture is another alternative therapy you might want to try. Research has shown that it is beneficial in treating high blood pressure and has resulted in an improved quality of life in patients with breast cancer who are taking an anti-estrogen treatment.[22] Plus, the simple act of having to lie still in a quiet place during an acupuncture session gives you a chance to decompress.

Break Down Your Fears

Sometimes the biggest things—paying for something major, like a college education or house; finding a new job; initiating a divorce— feel so insurmountable that it's hard to find the momentum to tackle them. So instead, you just stress about them. Make a list of the things you fear most and tackle the top items on your list.

Topping my list is financing my children's educations; I broke it down with these more doable tasks:

1. Look online to find resources and suggestions for setting up savings accounts, student loan options, and finding schools with excellent financial aid packages.

2. Meet with a certified financial analyst/college consultant to get my financial paperwork in order well in advance of the time I will be filling out financial aid forms.

3. Encourage friends and family members who would otherwise be purchasing birthday/graduation/confirmation gifts for my child to contribute to their college savings fund instead.

4. Involve my children in the process. Encourage them to save, minimize unnecessary spending, and understand the importance and cost of their college education.

Laughter Yoga

Megan, a forty-one-year-old research assistant, found herself in an emotional rut after a divorce and a move to a new city. She started experiencing daily stress headaches and was unable to sleep through the night. She thought that things would improve once she was settled in her new apartment, but three months later, she still felt sad and alone.

One evening, she walked past a local health club and noticed a sign for a laughter yoga class. She decided to give it a try. The discipline, if you can give it that hard-edged term, started in 1995, and there are now classes in over sixty countries worldwide. Based on the fact that the body doesn't know the difference between fake and real laughter, the classes, which combine laughing for no apparent reason with yogic breathing, use various playful tactics to get students laughing contagiously.

Megan left the first class with a sense of unexpected calm, and for the first time since her move, felt warmth and compassion from soon-to-be friends in the class. She almost immediately noticed an improvement in her overall outlook, as well as a decrease in her insomnia and headaches. She felt so good, she actually convinced several of her coworkers to join the class. They've been laughing ever since.

For more information on laughter yoga, check out www.laughter yoga.org.

Laugh Often and Fully

The potential benefits of giggling include improvement in immune function, a better tolerance for pain, and fewer responses to stress. Laughing is like yawning: it's contagious. So make an effort to be around people you find funny; watch comedies; spend time with a child (if you don't have one, borrow one from a friend or relative for the day); take a laughter yoga class, which is a favorite of the HAPPY Heart crowd (see sidebar, page 111). Beatrice, one of the HAPPY Heart participants, dances around the house nightly with her husband. "We pretend I'm a ballerina in the Boston ballet," she says with a laugh. "He acts like he's lifting me up, and we laugh. We do the tango, we sing. We just get really silly." I saw a bumper sticker on the way home from work one afternoon, and I wish I had one for myself. It read, "She who laughs lasts."

Three Easy First Steps Across the Stress Management Bridge

1. **Declutter your bedroom.** If you're like most people, you likely have stacks of books, clothes, shoes, dust bunnies, and other random piles strewn around your bedroom, which doesn't create the most restful, relaxing environment. A good standard for a healthy bedroom comes from health coach Slicis: "Would you allow a friend or family member to recover from an illness in your bedroom?" she asks. "If not, why do you think it's good for you to sleep there night after night?"

2. **Prepare for worst-case scenarios.** Make extra keys for your house and car and put them in a safe place (not in your house or car, obviously). Make extra copies of your birth and marriage certificates, passport, insurance papers, social security card, will, and any other important papers and put them in a fireproof safe. Copy your drivers license and all your credit cards so you'll have that information in case your wallet gets stolen. Minimizing the aftermath when things go wrong can substantially lower stress levels.

3. **Make a to-do list weekly or daily.** Doing so helps you prioritize what you need to get done in a certain period of time. There is something very rewarding about checking off the list task by task. The simple act of crossing something out eases your stress and your worry about falling behind.

chapter five

The Exercise Bridge

At age forty-five, Heather hardly ever left her house, or, unfortunately, even her bedroom. Obese and suffering from lupus and scleroderma, two autoimmune diseases, she basically lay in bed for five years. "All I did was feel sorry for myself, and think, 'poor me, poor me,'" she says. The only time she cheered up was when her three grandkids came to visit her, but even then, she was embarrassed that they had to see her in such a depressing state. The few times she did get out into the fresh air was for medical appointments. She desperately needed new knees, but her doctor was concerned her ailing body might not make it through the surgery. "I'd rather die on the operating table trying to get better than live like this anymore," she responded.

Thankfully, Heather survived the operation. The two new knees gave her a fresh start, but they were by no means a guarantee of success. I have watched many patients benefit from a hip replacement, an improved heart, or other surgical procedures, but fail to make the lasting changes necessary to actually capitalize on the second chance medical technology has given them. Desperate not to take two steps back, Heather made a purchase that guaranteed she couldn't revert back to her lounge-all-day habits. "I got a dog to make me walk every day," she says with a laugh, "She's my motivation and my soul mate." These days, the pair walks at least a mile a day, and Heather often goes farther than her furry companion can go. "I have a carriage for her, because she gets lazy and I want to keep going," she says. "I like to challenge myself." I fully endorse Heather's furry strategy to stay motivated. I often tell my patients I would love to be able to write a prescription to get a dog. Owning a dog that needs to be walked daily ensures that the owner will get regular exercise. Plus, canines make a nearly perfect companion: they listen without judgment, never talk back, and love unconditionally.

But Heather does more than just push Bella, her Lhasa apso, in the stroller. She and her grandchildren are now Nintendo Wii devotees, playing baseball, tiptoeing across an imaginary wire, and bowling. "My grandson always beats me at boxing," she says. "The kids laugh at me, and I laugh right along with them," she says. During the summer, the two generations ride bikes together, and Heather leads her granddaughter's friends in impromptu water aerobics classes. In addition, Heather regularly attends several classes the HAPPY Heart program offers, including stretch and relax, which is a hybrid of yoga and strength training, tai chi, and Zumba, a Latin dance–inspired aerobics workout.

Now weighing sixty pounds less than when I first met her, Heather isn't just physically lighter. Her body and spirit seem as new as her knees. Her cardiac-related stats have improved significantly as have her symptoms from lupus and scleroderma. While she is not entirely symptom free, she is now able to do anything she wants without pain. It's hard to believe this quick-to-laugh, charismatic woman was ready to be done with life just a few years ago. Now her life couldn't be fuller. When she's not working or spending time with friends, she's walking, stretching, or dancing. The only time her head hits the pillow is when the moon is up. "I fall asleep in minutes," she says with a smile.

The Physical Benefits of Exercise

Heather has discovered firsthand the myriad benefits exercise can bring to one's body, and you can too.

You'll Lose Weight

When you move with intention, you burn more calories than you do at rest and, as a result, are more likely to lose weight. The connection is a no-brainer, but the end result—a BMI in the healthy range—is invaluable to every part of your body from your knees to your ovaries. Think about how you feel when you have to carry two bags of groceries up a flight of stairs: those extra twenty pounds make your heart beat faster, your breath quicken, and your muscles ache. The effort is much harder than if you weren't carrying anything. When those twenty (or more) pounds are on your person, you obviously can't put them down; your body is continuously working on overdrive simply to function.

If you carry around an excessive amount of weight, your joints, especially those from your hips on down, are significantly strained, which can lead to degenerative joint disease (and the need for new knees, like Heather required). Aching joints make you less likely to want to exercise, so it becomes a vicious cycle: you need to move to lose weight and ease the burden on your joints, but they hurt so much, it doesn't seem possible. Obesity also increases the risk of many diseases, including cardiovascular disease, diabetes, endometrial cancer, breast cancer, and cervical cancer. What's more, if you're obese and want to become pregnant, studies show that you'll have a harder time becoming pregnant—and if you do, you run the risk of having more complications than a woman with a healthier weight.[1]

You'll Have a Longer Life

According to the U.S. Department of Health and Human Services, people who exercise seven hours a week have a 40 percent lower chance of dying early compared to those who do less than thirty minutes a week.[2] If an hour a day feels like a huge commitment, realize that simply walking for two hours a week is also associated with a significantly lower risk of mortality; in fact, the biggest improvement in mortality rates that the Department tracked was seen between the categories of less than thirty minutes a week to ninety minutes weekly.[3] Translation: Moving between thirty and ninety minutes a week gives you the most drastic decrease in mortality.

Importantly, that improvement crosses all categories of size from average weight to obese. In other words, if you're overweight, you don't have to downsize before you're able to enjoy the health benefits. Get moving, and they'll naturally accrue.

You'll Enjoy a Better Quality of Life

Although it's natural to need help from people in all stages of life, having to rely on somebody to help you out of bed or do your grocery shopping simply because you haven't kept your body in a capable state is beyond frustrating. I see patients regularly who can't walk from room to room in a small house or out to the mailbox because of pains in their joints, shortness of breath, and overall fatigue. Exercise boosts your bones, muscles, and organs so that you have natural strength to complete everyday tasks—and more importantly, participate in life. "I have more energy than I had before I started exercising," says Maria, one of my patients who started going to the gym four or five times weekly about two years ago. "I feel like I can do anything."

You'll Build a Stronger, Less Disease-Prone Heart

The heart is a muscle, just like your quads or your biceps, and the more you challenge it through exercise, the stronger it gets. Exercise and its effects on the heart have been a research and clinical interest of mine over the past decade, and I've been involved with some ground-breaking studies. In one that focused on collegiate rowers, a team of colleagues and I found that exercise enlarges the heart cavities. Larger cavities allow the heart to pump a higher volume of blood in a more efficient manner. As a result, muscles and organs reap the benefits because they receive a more voluminous flow of oxygen-rich blood.[4]

A similar study focused on middle-aged rowers and illustrated another helpful by-product of exercise: relaxed blood vessels.[5] As we age, the heart muscle and blood vessels naturally stiffen and become less flexible; blood vessels tend toward the feel of an inflexible piece of peanut brittle instead of pliant taffy. Relaxed blood vessels contribute to lower blood pressure and a decreased likelihood of developing plaque along the arterial walls.

Finally, all the markers of a healthy heart—blood pressure, LDL (bad) cholesterol, HDL (good) cholesterol, markers of inflammation—are influenced in a positive way through movement.

Your Heart Won't Know If You're Thirty-Five or Sixty-Five

Not only does regular exercise return your heart to a healthier state, it maintains it at a level that defies aging. One study, based at the University of Texas Southwestern Medical Center, compared the heart relaxation function (HRF)—the period when the heart isn't pumping blood—of twelve senior athletes, average age sixty-eight, with fourteen younger, but sedentary people, average age twenty-eight. HRF is one of the first cardiac characteristics to unfavorably change when the heart declines, so it's a great indication of heart health. When HRF is normal, the heart can fill with blood efficiently, with a minimal effort. In the study, both groups had similar HRFs. So in effect, the almost seventy-year-olds were as heart healthy as people forty years younger![6]

What's more, even if you have already have had complications or issues with your heart, research indicates exercise improves nearly any situation. One study out of Emory University focused on thirty-two women, ages fifty to eighty-five, with abnormal HRF due to excessive stiffening of the heart muscle. Half of the group participated in a three-month walking program, while the other half simply received education about exercise. At the end of the study, the women who were on the walking program were able to go farther and faster than the other half and were more inclined to stick with exercise.[7] Although scientists didn't focus on the heart muscle directly, the results they saw suggest an improvement in the group's underlying HRF impairment.

You'll Build a Stronger, Less Disease-Prone Body

The laundry list of diseases that exercise can either prevent or minimize includes the following:

- **Osteoporosis.** Researchers at the University of Padova in Italy looked at 125 postmenopausal women, the age group to which osteoporosis is most threatening. They put fifty-eight of the women on an exercise program that included strength training, cardiovascular conditioning, balance exercises, and joint mobility moves. The other sixty-seven women did not exercise. In eleven months, the group that moved improved their bone mass scores—an indication of osteoporosis—significantly as well as their overall physical capacity. The bone quality of the group that didn't move decreased in that same span of time.[8]

- **Diabetes.** Experts from Virginia Tech University performed a detailed analysis of studies that involved resistance training (lifting weights) and preventing diabetes in middle- to older-aged adults. They reviewed 142 studies and determined that strength training improves the ability of insulin to move more glucose into a cell, leaving less insulin and glucose in the bloodstream. High insulin levels are a sign of diabetes. In addition, it decreases the amount of abdominal fat while simultaneously improving lean muscle mass, both factors involved in the development of diabetes.[9]

- **Fibromyalgia.** Two studies in Europe, one in Spain and one in Sweden, both found that regular exercise improves pain levels and physical function in women with fibromyalgia— a series of symptoms that involves chronic pain, fatigue, multiple tender points, sleep disturbance, and psychological distress.[10]

- **Breast cancer.** A Canadian paper looked at the results of seventy-three breast cancer and exercise-related studies and concluded that active women have 25 percent less of a chance of contracting breast cancer than their sedentary counterparts.

(Among the strongest positive associations were women who exercised regularly after menopause, reinforcing that it's never too late to start.)[11]

- **Inflammation.** A study out of the University of Minnesota followed 319 inactive women, ages eighteen to thirty, who were a mix of underweight, normal weight, and overweight. For sixteen weeks, half were put on an exercise plan and the other half didn't change their routines. The exercise group saw a significant reduction in their C-reactive protein levels (the protein described earlier that is released by the liver and has been associated with increased inflammation and risk of heart disease). The biggest reductions were seen in the heaviest women, which illustrates how beneficial and important exercise is, no matter what the number on the scale says. "These findings suggest that adopting an exercise routine early in life may decrease future risk of breast cancer and other chronic diseases in obese women," conclude the authors.[12]

You'll Sleep Better

You might feel the biggest benefit of today's workout when you wake up tomorrow morning, feeling rested and ready for the day. Investigators from Northwestern University studied seventeen sedentary adults with chronic insomnia, putting half on an aerobic exercise program of moderate intensity and leaving half with no intervention. After sixteen weeks, the group that sweated regularly greatly improved the quality and duration of their sleep, overall mood, and feeling of tiredness during the day.[13] I can't stress how important these results are; as mentioned above, poor sleep habits are associated with increased risk of anxiety, depression, cardiovascular disease, obesity, and diabetes.

The Mental Benefits of Exercise

Heather's mind benefited as much as her body did from her newly active lifestyle; the mental gains from exercise are as invaluable as the physical ones.

You'll Feel Less Stress

Moving your body boosts your mood. Walking and running are a kind of meditation in motion. The rhythm of your steps takes your mind off a demanding boss or overflowing to-do list. Activities that require more focus, like playing tennis or tai chi, force you to concentrate on the motion so you have to stay in the moment. Either way, you end a session of exercise feeling more settled and content—and less stressed.

Research bears this out. The Ochsner Clinic Foundation in New Orleans investigated how stress is affected by exercise. Fifty-three cardiac patients who had high levels of stress were offered twelve weeks of exercise classes: a ten-minute warm-up; thirty to forty minutes of walking, rowing, or other aerobic exercise; and a ten-minute cooldown. They took the group class three times a week and then were asked to exercise on their own one to three times a week. Comparing the results with a group of cardiac patients who didn't exercise but had similar stress levels, the active ones reduced their stress levels considerably. In addition, they were 60 percent less likely to die in the following six years.[14]

Similarly, if you're prone to anxiety, exercise can help diffuse those feelings too. Scientists at the University of Georgia analyzed the results of forty studies that involved three thousand patients with a variety of diseases, including heart disease, multiple sclerosis, and cancer. Those who exercised regularly reported a 20 percent reduction in anxiety symptoms compared to those who remained sedentary.[15]

You Will Be Less Prone to Depression

Exercise releases endorphins and other feel-good chemicals that simultaneously make you happier, decrease sensations of pain, and lead to more organized, cohesive thought. What's more, the simple act of sweating (which increases your core body temperature) may simply feel soothing.

Over the past three decades, doctors have extensively studied patients with depression, conducting studies that compare the effects of taking an antidepressant with those of exercise. The results regularly point to exercise having a similar effect as an antidepressant. A recent study, the SMILE study (Standard Medical Intervention and Long-term Exercise, conducted at Duke University), further solidified the connection. Studying 202 sedentary adults with major depressive disorder, doctors put half on an exercise program, a quarter on Zoloft, and a quarter on a placebo. Four months after the study began, they found that the regular exercisers had similar results as those on medication. Following up with the patients a year later, the researchers found even more encouraging results. The exercisers had 60 percent more people who had recovered from depression, compared to the medication group, which had a relapse rate of six times more than the exercise group.[16]

Aerobic exercise isn't the only kind of activity that lessens depression. Another study, performed at the Boston University School of Medicine, looked at the effects of yoga on gamma-aminobutyric acid (GABA) levels in the brain; low levels are associated with depression and anxiety. They found that those who did sixty minutes of yoga had a 27 percent increase in GABA levels, compared to those who spent that hour quietly reading.[17]

You'll Have an Enhanced Sense of Self-Esteem

Exercise can, in essence, be broken down into two parts: setting goals and seeing results. The simple act of setting an achievable goal—losing ten pounds, walking for an hour—and then taking steps toward meeting it can make you flush with confidence. Your clothes fit better, you have more energy, and your mood is lighter. With some further effort and dedication, you meet your goal, which causes your confidence to blossom even more.

Just ask my patient Maggie, who is a mother of two school-aged kids and a busy interior designer. She was referred to me because of her shortness of breath. Twenty-five pounds overweight with a staggering blood pressure of 170/100, she was a ticking time bomb. A former runner, she stopped exercising when she became a mom. Not making eye contact as she spoke to me, she used the common excuse that she was just too busy to do anything about it. We had an honest talk and I could tell she understood how serious her situation was.

A year later, she had dropped the extra weight by working out four days a week, alternating between the elliptical machine and walking on the treadmill. She logged a normal blood pressure. While her numbers are important, what was more startling was how she carried herself. I could see she found great pride in making herself a priority again; she didn't grow taller, but she certainly stood taller. I saw it in Maggie and I see it in my HAPPY Heart patients. Once they know they're taking care of themselves and they feel the results, a quiet confidence envelopes them.

Your Brain Will Be More Nimble

The increased blood flow that hits all your muscles also heads to your brain, which keeps the blood vessels in the brain relaxed and also produces brain-derived neurotrophic factor, which fosters the creation and growth of brain cells.

Multiple studies have shown that people who exercise regularly have a reduced risk of Alzheimer's and other cognitive disorders, and other studies have determined that aerobic exercise enhances memory and brain function. Wanting to investigate the effect of resistance training, researchers at the University of British Columbia put 106 women, ages sixty-five to seventy-five, on a strength-training program either once or twice a week for thirty-minute sessions. The eight-move program included exercises for the major muscle groups, like leg presses, bicep curls, and hamstring curls. After a year, both groups improved their *cognitive function* (the ability to reason, organize, and decide) by 10 to 12 percent, while a control group, which did balance and tone training (read: not as intense exercise) lost 0.5 percent of their cognitive function.[18] I find this study to be very exciting; as little as thirty minutes weekly of resistance training doesn't just make your body stronger—it makes your mind stronger too.

Safe and Healthy Exercise

Before you exercise, here are a few important guidelines:

- In 2008, the U.S. Department of Health and Human Services issued comprehensive guidelines for improved health. They recommend at least 150 minutes of exercise at a moderate intensity or 75 minutes of exercise at a vigorous intensity— or a combination of the two—weekly. For additional health benefits, like weight loss and improved cardiovascular capacity, increase the amounts to 300 minutes of moderate exercise or 150 minutes of vigorous movement.[19]

- If you're coming from little or no activity, the guidelines suggest you "start low and go slow."[20] Gradually increase the intensity and duration of your exercise program.

- If you have any concerns about your heart or any other part of your body, talk to your physician before you begin.

- If you are a heart attack survivor, consult your cardiologist to enroll in a cardiac rehabilitation program prior to starting a self-directed exercise regimen. Your entry into exercise should be gradual and supervised. If you develop any new symptoms with exercise, be sure to have them checked out immediately. But don't be intimidated to start moving. Despite the fact that cardiac rehabilitation reduces risk of death after a heart attack, only 30 percent of heart attack survivors take part in these programs.[21] What's more disheartening to me, though, is that women are much less likely than men to do so.

- If you have joint or mobility issues, try getting in a pool. Swimming or taking a water aerobics class provides the same benefits as exercising on land does, but the water provides a forgiving, supportive medium in which to move your body without impacting your joints.

- If you are pregnant and healthy, but have not been active prior to becoming pregnant, aim for 150 minutes of weekly moderate activity. If you were a regular gym-goer, you can keep up your routine as long as you discuss it with your doctor first. Remember that your tendons become more relaxed with pregnancy and your balance may be affected by weight gain, so be sure to err on the side of caution. If you're going to run or do something similarly intense, please heed the current guidelines, which recommend that you exercise at an intensity that allows you to talk while doing aerobic exercise.[22]

- If you have a disability or chronic condition, you should discuss with your health care provider what amounts and types of exercise are appropriate for your situation.

Building the Bridge to Exercise

While two new knees and four little paws definitely contributed to Heather's success on her path to a healthy lifestyle, there are a couple key components of her story that can help anybody embrace exercise.

Go at a Comfortable Pace

Heather hardly ever changes into traditional exercise clothes to walk or do a class. So many people think exercise needs to be an all-out, red-cheeked, sweaty effort that requires a gym membership, special clothes, and huge chunks of time. While that's one way to get it done, there are plenty of other more moderate ways that will still let your body and mind enjoy the bounty exercise has to offer. "Put on music and dance around the house as you vacuum," says Donna Slicis. "You don't have to be suffering in a gym to be active." Many of the studies cited above used walking as exercise, which is a great place to start. It's a simple motion you already know how to do, and you just need shoes and a direction to go in.

Be Realistic About What You Can Handle

Heather's body is in a place where short walks and sessions of Wii are perfect for her. Coming out of a sedentary lifestyle, setting overly ambitious goals can be a recipe for failure. "People often come to me and say, 'I'm going to exercise an hour for five days a week,'" says Susan Lane, RN, MSN, MBA, a yoga and tai chi instructor with HAPPY Heart. "I say, 'Great that you have those goals, but let's start smaller: can you walk up a flight of stairs a day?' They say sure, so we begin there." Lane realizes that's not enough activity, but, like me, she'd rather have a patient complete something little every day than attempt something so big that it feels impossible to start. The small, doable tasks not only get your body headed in the right direction, but they also force you to consciously find time in your day to move. Most importantly, they let you taste success.

Fortunately, just like exercise doesn't have to be a marathonesque effort to start, it also doesn't require you to be all-in to receive the good it can bring into your life. In other words, you can dip your toe in the (sweaty) water without having to jump into the lake, and you can still improve your health. A goal of two to two-and-a-half hours of moderate exercise a week is hugely beneficial to your overall well-being. That's four or five thirty-minute walks a week, a goal you can incrementally work toward. Broken down that way, it doesn't feel so intimidating. It also doesn't have to be in one consecutive session. Research has shown that breaking up, say, a forty-minute walk into two twenty-minute walks doesn't forfeit the key health benefits.

Finally, although weight loss is a goal for many people, don't let the number on the scale decide success for you. Being physically fit and still carrying a few extra pounds is much preferable to being unfit and overweight. In a study, published in the *American Heart Journal* in early 2011, doctors followed 855 men and women, all of whom had suffered a heart attack or had severe heart problems, for fourteen years. Using data from treadmill tests, they found that fit but overweight patients were twice as likely to die as their thin, fit counterparts, and fit and obese patients were three times as likely to die. Sounds bad, but consider this: unfit people with normal weights were *ten* times more likely to die.[23] "The bottom line is that fitness modulates the prognosis in patients with coronary artery disease according to their body weight," Dr. Francisco Lopez-Jiminez, a heart specialist and study leader, told *Reuters Health*.[24]

Mix It Up

Dabbling in everything from belly dancing to water aerobics, Heather also mixes up the way she moves, which keeps both her body and mind fresh. If you have an activity you love to do, certainly there's nothing wrong with focusing on that. But if you swim, walk, strength-train, and do yoga all in one week, your body and mind will be challenged in different ways—a good thing, because your muscles will stay strong and pliable, and your mind won't have a chance to be bored. It goes without saying, though, that any activity you do should be something you enjoy. If you're forcing yourself to "love" swimming, even though you may gaze longingly at the racquetball courts as you walk to the pool, you're inevitably going to give swimming up. Instead, pick up your racquet and have at it.

Buddy Up

When people ask me for the one piece of workout equipment they should get, I don't say a treadmill or a set of weights. It's a workout buddy. A friend or neighbor or sister who is in a place similar to where you are now (it's not fun to be chasing after somebody constantly or always feel like you're being held back), has a schedule that is similar to the one you have, and wants to meet the same goals you do. It may take a little effort on your part to find her—good places to start include a class at a YMCA or a local walking or running club—but, like exercise, the work is definitely worth it.

Heather is rarely alone when she's exercising: she plays with her grandkids, she walks with her dog, she cha-chas to Latin rhythms with girlfriends. When we poll our HAPPY Heart participants about what they like most about the program, the most popular answer every time is the group dynamic. "I love my girls," says Heather, referring to her fellow participants. "They make everything feel so much easier." Making a standing exercise date with a friend is invaluable: you may allow yourself to skip a walk, but you won't stand up a friend who is waiting for you on the corner. Once you meet her, the minutes go by so much faster with conversation and laughter.

As a lifelong runner who has passed many miles on the road with great women, I, along with plenty of other women, can testify that the friendships you solidify during exercise sessions tend to be some of the strongest and most reliable ones going.

Try Not to Overthink It

Bella the dog needs to walk, so there is no choice. Heather gets on her shoes and walks too. "So often people fixate on exercise, telling themselves I don't feel like it today or I don't want to do it," says Lane. "You don't give yourself that runaround when you brush your teeth." Exercise is just like brushing your teeth: nonnegotiable self-maintenance. "Make the activity doable, and then go do it," she says. "Don't give yourself a choice."

Realize You May Be Uncomfortable

There's a reason why most people don't exercise: it's not always pleasant. But often, motion—and increased blood flow—helps injuries heal. (That's why, after a surgery, patients are often encouraged to get up and walk around.) Katherine, a HAPPY Heart participant, had to use a cane because of the arthritis in her left foot. Through yoga, stretching, and dancing in Zumba, she found that, as she says, "The more I use my foot, the less it hurts. It hurts initially when I get going, but in the long run, I know it's helping." These days, she's walking without a cane.

Sweat, Strength-Train, or Both?

Exercise comes in two varieties: aerobic and strength. Aerobic is generally anything that gets your heart rate up, like brisk walking, swimming, or tennis, while strength is concentrated on building muscular strength through resistance, like lifting weights. You don't really isolate one system, though, when you exercise. For instance, if you're doing a weight circuit that focuses on your primary muscles, your heart rate will rise as you do squats and push-ups. Similarly, if you're doing a StairMaster, your heart will be working hard, but your lower body muscles will also be building strength.

Confused about where to start? If you're coming from a mostly sedentary life, here are some of the suggestions I often give my patients:

- **Walking.** Try it because it's accessible, can easily be done while chatting with a friend, and offers fresh air.
- **Zumba or another low-impact aerobics class.** Try it because it's high on group motivation and great music, plus it's a chance to try something new.

- **Aqua aerobics.** Try it because it's easy on the joints, and the water offers extra resistance for building strength.
- **Tai chi.** Try it because it's a connection between the body and mind, improves balance and coordination, and allows you to tap into the unlimited supply of *qi* (internal energy).
- **Cycling outside or inside on a stationary bike.** Try it because it's low-impact, so it won't hurt your joints, and you can cover a lot of ground in a little time.

If you're unable to start with any of those activities, some of my HAPPY Heart patients begin in a chair, with chair yoga, chair Zumba, and chair strength training. Remember that all movement is good movement.

If you're already moderately active, you might like these options:

- **Brisk walking or running.** Up the challenge by adding intervals (short bursts of speed) to your workouts.
- **Swimming.** Up the challenge by learning all four strokes.
- **Tennis.** Up the challenge by joining a league and competing.
- **Doing the elliptical or StairMaster at the gym.** Up the challenge by increasing the length of your workout sessions or increasing the level for interval work.
- **Strength training.** Twice a week, everybody should also do some form of strength training (it can be counted toward the weekly exercise goal of 150 minutes). Lifting weights make your body more capable of performing daily tasks, but also, muscle burns more calories than fat, so the more muscle you build, the more calories your body will burn when you are at rest. A simple routine that hits all your major muscles is sufficient. You can take a class at a gym, do a DVD at home with some hand weights, or find exercises online that fit your level.

Heed the Rule of Eighteen

A health coach I heard speak at a woman's heart event years ago mentioned that if you do any activity for eighteen days in a row, it will become ingrained in your head. To streamline the process, make a chart with the numbers one to eighteen on it, then get up and move: walk, dance, do yoga, whatever you feel like doing that day. Cross off the number when you do it. After eighteen days, exercise, which was previously an unpleasant, easily avoided activity, will feel like an essential part of your life.

Set a Goal

It should be attainable, not over the top. If you're new to walking, maybe it's walking a five-kilometer course (3.1 miles) for a charity. If you're headed to a wedding, maybe it's losing five pounds so you can look great in your sundress. You can also have a bigger goal, like running a marathon or losing fifty pounds, looming in the background, but taking small, tangible steps—lose five pounds in two months or do a five-kilometer run in three months—is the way to accomplish them. Amy, one of the HAPPY Heart patients, has a fun goal of running on the beach as she flies a kite. To get there, she's walking regularly and working on pushing her pace so she can keep that kite aloft.

Get Feedback

If you're embarking on an exercise routine, write down your weight and your waist circumference at its smallest point. (If you're discouraged with your numbers, know that the average American woman, according to the CDC, is almost 5'4", almost 165 pounds, and has a waist circumference of 37 inches.[25]) If you're not up for seeing numbers, skip the scale and use a strategy we use at HAPPY Heart: use a string to measure your waist. Mark your circumference on the string and then put it in a safe place. Either way, take your measurements again in two to three months.

Record It

About that log you just wrote your numbers in: learn to use it. Write down what exercise you did, how long you did it, and anything else you'd like to remember about your workout. (You felt great; your knee hurt; you didn't want to go but were so glad you did.) When you record your data, you're more likely to stick with the program; tangibly seeing your progress is priceless when your motivation wanes.

Three Easy First Steps Across the Exercise Bridge

1. Call a friend and schedule a month's worth of exercise sessions—walks, classes at the gym, whatever you both enjoy—together.

2. Make a new playlist for your workouts; research shows that listening to music makes exercise feel easier.[26] Not up for mindless tunes? Download a podcast or a book (many public libraries have them available for free).

3. If you're going to exercise at home, clear out a designated space. (The more light and open space there is, the better.) Give yourself ample room for movement and pull together all the equipment you may need. Suggestions include hand

weights, a jump rope, resistance bands, a Swiss ball, and a television if you're going to do videos. If you find you enjoy working out at home, consider investing in a treadmill or elliptical machine.

chapter six

The Nutrition Bridge

Laurie, now sixty-two years old, quit smoking in her thirties. Obviously this was a great move for her health, but she, like many people, traded cigarettes for chips, cookies, and other junk food. The pounds piled on slowly but surely, and Laurie decided dieting was the way to go. "I've tried them all: the cabbage soup diet, the red diet, the grapefruit diet," she ticks off. "I didn't do Atkins, because I thought that was foolish, but I have tried to fast." Not surprisingly, nothing worked because diets don't work for the long term. Some weight came off temporarily, but more always returned.

An avid reader, Laurie is well versed in the nuts and bolts of nutrition. For instance, she knows why you should eat breakfast: it fires up your metabolism for the day and promotes the eating of three balanced meals, not one or two huge ones. But knowledge and action are two very different things. "I'm not hungry when I get up," she explains. "I just have no interest in breakfast." She rarely takes a bite before 10 a.m., which is actually an early start for her. Her cupboards house containers and containers of oatmeal, a solid breakfast choice, but she has never cracked one open. "I am going to do it one day," she says. I hope she will, but I am not so sure it'll happen. Eating patterns are some of the most difficult to change.

No woman I know has an uncomplicated relationship with food. Far from just being the sustenance our bodies need to function, food plays a multitude of roles in our lives. It comforts us when we're lonely. It brings us together to celebrate or to grieve. It fills the gaps when we're bored. It fills us up when we're down. It connects us with friends and family. It provides us with a way to nurture our family and friends. "Ninety percent of the time I am putting food in my mouth for a reason other than hunger," Laurie says matter-of-factly (and correctly). And when you widen the lens to include what we eat, things get much more complex. A person's finances, the effect of the media, the time of year and of day, patterns of childhood, and plenty of other intangible yet very real influences come into the picture as well.

Instead of letting her rational side rule her appetite, Laurie often lets her diet be dominated by emotions. A single adoptive foster parent and a former social worker, Laurie is a helper who likes to reach out to other people and make their lives better. Severe arthritis in her knees and hands forced her to prematurely retire from the job she loved. In addition, her adult son, along with his family, moved out of state. When the two anchoring things to which she devoted her energy disappeared, she filled the holes in her life with food. "I've always been a person who has had control," she explains, "and now I have nothing to control. I don't work, my son isn't close by—I wasn't a controlling parent, but you know what I mean—and that's one of the biggest reasons why I eat."

That explanation doesn't hit on her inability to eat breakfast, but I admire her for being able to dissect the issues around most of her consumption, something that is terribly difficult for many people. Self-awareness is an important step toward managing how and what you eat.

Emotional Eating

Feeling desperate and lonely, Vanessa sat in her bed one night and ate a six-pack of Klondike ice cream bars. Coming home after a long day, Katie had a dinner that consisted of half of a hunk of salami, half of a block of cheese, and a bag of crackers. Both of these women are HAPPY Heart participants, but the notion of eating way too much because of sadness, stress, or some other negative emotion is something to which most of us can relate. Who hasn't stood in front of a refrigerator with the door open for too long, looking for something sweet or fatty to eat, hoping it will temporarily ease the pain, decrease the stress, or soothe the mind?

This isn't news to you, but food can't do those things. Food can't fill a void, bring back a loved one, or make you feel accepted. There's a reason why people who are going to undergo gastric bypass are required to have counseling before they enter the operating room; if they don't take time to analyze their unhealthy relationship with food prior to needing to alter it, the surgical procedure can't help. Melanie Pearsall, RD, LDN, CDE, the nutritionist on the HAPPY Heart team, often reminds people considering such surgery that it is not surgery on the brain, but your brain will have to change as much as your stomach has. In fact, after gastric bypass, many patients actually report going through a tough adjustment phase after losing their closest friend: an unending supply of food.

Research suggests that food can often be a coping mechanism. An American Psychological Association study of almost 1,800 people found that over 48 percent overeat or eat unhealthy foods because of stress. What's more, another 39 percent have skipped a meal because of stress, a situation that can easily lead to overeating; when you deprive yourself, you have a tendency to go overboard later.[1] British researchers analyzed the food habits and feelings of nearly two thousand students in their first year at University, when intense demands, a new environment, and a lack of familiar social support can cause a great deal of stress. They found a significant association between increased levels of stress and depression and increased consumption of sweets and fast foods, as well as decreased consumption of healthy foods like fruits and vegetables.[2]

Wanting to detail food selections under stress, scientists out of Montclair State University in New Jersey put out of bowls of grapes, M&M's, peanuts, and potato chips, and then gave seventeen participants easy anagrams (word puzzles) to solve, another seventeen participants unsolvable anagrams, and let them eat whatever they wanted as they worked on their problems. The people with the easy puzzles ate 15 grams of grapes, while the ones with the difficult puzzles, who later reported feeling stressed about the situation, ate about 2 grams. The ratio was similarly inverted for M&M's: the stressed-out group ate nearly three times more chocolate bits than the relaxed group.[3]

Mindless Eating

Eating out of boredom can be just as harmful and can actually be more difficult to manage, since the opportunities for mindless eating are endless. (Same situation: the refrigerator is open, but this time you're looking for a morsel to eat while you pass the time in front of a television or computer.) Kristin, a HAPPY Heart participant, told us how she sat in front of her television and ate a loaf of bread with butter as she watched her favorite shows. In fact, several studies have discovered a definitive link between prolonged television watching and obesity in children, teens, and women. The renowned Nurses' Health Study looked at fifty thousand women aged thirty to fifty-five, and found that a woman's odds of obesity rose 23 percent and her risk of type 2 diabetes rose 14 percent for every additional two daily hours of television time she logged.[4]

Another study, published in the *Journal of the American College of Cardiology*, concluded that time spent in front of a television screen was associated with higher levels of the inflammatory marker C-reactive protein, lower levels of the beneficial form of HDL cholesterol, and higher body mass index. What was interesting is that the association remained even when the level of physical activity was considered; in other words, people who exercised had similar results to those who didn't regularly sweat.[5] One possible reason for the findings: time in front of the screen is often spent with a bowl of chips, a can of soda or beer, or other unhealthy snacks.

Building the Bridge to Better Nutrition

Laurie, like all of us, is a work in progress. "I don't think I'll ever be thin," she says, "but I am making a conscious effort to make life changes. I could be doing a lot better, I'm sure, but I'm trying not to eat when I'm stressed or upset." That is all I can ask: Be cognizant of your eating patterns. Think about why and what you're eating.

This chapter in *Smart at Heart* is the only time I'll ask you to think less with your heart and more with your head. Why? Because your approach to eating and your relationship with food can define your physical health. Although you can cook out of love and affection, you need to make smart choices about what you cook—and how much and why you eat. At the end of the day, food by itself cannot nourish your heart or spirit; it can only provide you with the fuel your body needs to get you through the day. You eat to live, not live to eat. When you think of food as fuel, it's easier to step away from the chocolate cake, not hit the drive-thru at McDonald's, and make healthier choices overall. I'm not saying you can't enjoy all types of food or eat food in a celebratory manner; in fact, I want you to make an effort to savor every bite you take, whether it's an apple, french fry, or piece of wedding cake. What I am saying is that food can't solve an argument, squash unpleasant memories, or relieve depression. Using it in that manner can only backfire: not only do you feel physically unwell from consuming too much, but you also haven't dealt with the root of the problem, which will likely lead to more overeating.

In 2011, the AHA produced new dietary recommendations for the prevention of cardiovascular disease in women, which are what I suggest my patients follow.[6]

NUTRIENT	SERVING	SERVING SIZE EXAMPLES
Fruits and vegetables	$4^1/_2$ cups or more per day	• 1 cup raw leafy vegetable • $^1/_2$ cup cut-up raw or cooked vegetable • $^1/_2$ cup vegetable or fruit juice • 1 medium-sized fruit • $^1/_4$ cup dried fruit • $^1/_2$ cup fresh, frozen, or canned fruit
Fish	2 servings per week	• 3.5 oz. cooked (and preferably oily) fish, like salmon, herring, or mackerel
Fiber	30 g per day (look for 1.1 g of fiber for every 10 g of carbohydrates)	• Bran cereal (check the label, but generally around 12 g per serving) • Split peas, lentils, and other beans (1 cup has 10 to 16 g) • Raspberries (1 cup has 8 g) • Avocado (one whole fruit has about 13 g)

NUTRIENT	SERVING	SERVING SIZE EXAMPLES
Whole grains	3 servings per day	• 1 slice bread • 1 oz. dry cereal • $^1/_2$ cup cooked whole-grain rice, pasta, or cereal
Sugar	No more than five servings per week (and no more than 450 calories per week from sugar-sweetened beverages)	• 1 tablespoon sugar • 1 tablespoon jelly or jam • $^1/_2$ cup sorbet • 1 cup lemonade
Nuts, legumes, and seeds	Four or more servings per week	• $^1/_3$ cup or 1.5 oz. nuts (avoid macadamia and salted nuts) • 2 tablespoons peanut butter • 2 tablespoons or 0.5 oz. seeds • $^1/_2$ cup cooked legumes
Saturated fat	Less than 7 percent total intake per day	• Found in fried foods, fat on meat, chicken skins, packaged desserts, butter, cheese, sour cream
Cholesterol	Less than 150 mg per day	• Found in animal meats, organ meats, eggs
Alcohol	No more than one drink per day	• 4 oz. of wine • 12 oz. of beer • 1.5 oz. of 80-proof spirits • 1 oz. of 100-proof spirits
Sodium	No more than 1,500 mg per day	
Trans-fatty acids	0	

But food guides aren't helpful if you can't apply them to your everyday life and make them your own. Here are some strategies Pearsall and I have found to be effective and easy to execute.

Take Small Steps

Although I advocate cleaning out your cupboards and tossing the junk when you're ready to focus on nutrition, it's also important not to think in a pass-or-fail mentality. Instead, think of your path to better eating as a long staircase, with each step getting you closer to a healthier you. If you eat fast food or pizza four nights a week, one step can be to downsize that to twice a week. If you never eat breakfast, start with a step of eating cereal or toast twice a week. If you're trying to convert to whole-wheat pasta, make your first meal with a quarter of the new variety and three-quarters of your favorite kind and then slowly increase the ratio. If you are a red meat devotee, incrementally reduce your portion sizes. Small changes can add up surprisingly quickly, in terms of your body's health; don't underestimate them. Plus, successful small changes can increase your confidence to initiate other changes.

A Different Kind of Sub

Here are some substitutes that can instantly make you healthier.

INSTEAD OF	TRY
Sour cream	Nonfat yogurt
Butter	Olive oil
Creamy salad dressing	Balsamic vinegar and olive oil
Ramen/mac-and-cheese	Whole-grain pasta and tomato sauce
Soda	Flavored water
Sugar	Stevia
Red meat	Fish
Prepackaged snacks	Your own bags of nuts, veggies, or fruit
Meat seven days a week	One vegetarian main dish weekly
Frying	Steaming or sautéing

Get in Balance

One of the simplest ways to make sure you have a well-rounded meal is to use the balanced plate method. When you approach creating a meal, mentally divide your plate in half. Think about filling one half with fruits or vegetables. Split the other half in half; one quarter is lean protein, like chicken or fish, and one quarter is grains or starches, like pasta.

The balanced plate is an easy concept to grasp, especially when your meal consists of simple foods like a chicken breast, multigrain roll, and salad, but what happens when you have a more complex meal? Figure out the dominant food of the meal, and go from there. Beef stew would ideally be equal parts of meat and potatoes and dominated by vegetables. With lasagna, cheese gives you protein, the pasta gives you starch, but the tomato sauce definitely doesn't make up half the meal. So add a large serving of vegetables or salad on the side.

Breathe

When you're in the middle of a fight with your husband or have work deadlines that seem impossible to meet, try not to beeline for the Ben & Jerry's. If that has been a habit, I realize it may feel like I'm asking the impossible, but countless patients have shown me it can be done. When you're feeling balanced, identify three or four easily accessible things you can do to put some space between you and food when you want to emotionally eat. Here are a few ideas: walk around the block, take a shower, go to your bedroom and practice guided relaxation (see page 107). "You learned to eat when you're stressed," says Pearsall. "Now you have to teach your body to want something else."

Avoid the Supersize

These days, our dining landscape is dominated by Big Gulps and plates the size of hubcaps. This is one time it's cool not to be trendy. Downsize your dinnerware. A nine-inch plate is plenty big, according to Brian Wansink, PhD, author of *Mindless Eating*, who also scientifically proved that people pour more alcohol into a short, stout glass than a tall, thin one.[7] Order the smallest portion possible at restaurants—if you're still hungry when you finish, you can order more—and at home, aim to use smaller glasses, plates, and spoons. In addition, put away extra bread or salad plates; all the food you eat in one meal should fit on one plate.

Read the Price Tag

When you're grocery shopping, there are two bits of information you should pay attention to: the ingredient list and the label on packaged foods. "Combined, they're the equivalent of a price tag for the food you're eating," says Pearsall. "The cost of an item isn't just how much money you pay. It's also the price the food takes from or adds to your well-being." Often, the ninety-nine cents you pay for a bag of potato chips will extract a much bigger toll on your body. "Sometimes when I put a spoonful of ice cream in my mouth, I think, okay, what is happening inside me?" says Beatrice, a HAPPY Heart participant. "How will this affect me today, tomorrow, this year?"

- **Ingredients.** Ideally, an ingredient list should contain items you can recognize and pronounce. "Even though ice cream isn't the healthiest food, an ingredient list like the one for Breyer's ice cream is a good model," says Pearsall, noting that the vanilla flavor has only milk, cream, sugar, natural tara gum, and natural vanilla flavor. In addition, ingredient lists should be relatively short; the longer they get, the farther the food strays from its most natural state. Ingredients are listed in order by weight: if the first item is whole grain and the last item is salt, that means that the whole grain makes up the majority of the food, while salt is only a sliver. (You can confirm that when you read the label.) Finally, try to avoid products whose ingredients include the word *hydrogenated*, which refers to fats that have been chemically altered to improve shelf life but that also increase total and LDL (bad) cholesterol.

- **The label.** A food label has a wealth of information on it, if you know how to read one. First of all, take a look at the serving size. A serving size is the amount the manufacturer has deemed appropriate for one serving. As such, the numbers on the food label correspond to that amount of food. For instance, if a serving size on a box of oats and honey granola is two-thirds of a cup, all the other information given—230 calories, 6 g of fat, 14 g of sugar, 5 g of protein— is applicable to two-thirds of a cup.

  "There's a huge disconnect between serving size and portion," says Pearsall. A portion is the amount you eat. So if your portion is two cups of granola, you'd have to triple all those numbers to get the accurate nutritional data: 690 calories, 18 g of fat, 42 g of sugar, 15 g of protein.

Hold the Salt

The newest USDA guidelines, released in early 2011, recognize that people either with or prone to high blood pressure will benefit from limiting their salt intake. They call for 2,300 milligrams a day of sodium—about the amount in a teaspoon of salt—for the general population. For African-Americans, individuals with hypertension, diabetes, or chronic kidney disease, and individuals ages fifty-one and older, the recommended number is reduced to 1,500 milligrams daily.[8] The AHA doesn't think the USDA goes low enough, and suggests 1,500 milligrams for all Americans.[9]

That doesn't mean you have to retire your kitchen's salt shaker. In fact, most of the sodium we eat comes from processed foods or foods we eat in restaurants; salt and fat are easy and cheap ways to make food taste better. It does mean, however, that if you're in a high-risk category, you need to be ultravigilant about your salt consumption, which means studying labels and limiting how often you eat out. Simply put, salt is toxic when it hits your bloodstream. If you're prone to high blood pressure or have other conditions that aggravate your blood pressure, too much salt can increase your blood pressure immediately, sometimes to a level that requires a visit to the ER. There are much less dangerous ways to make food taste better.

Get Familiar with Serving Sizes

What you consider an appropriate serving is likely larger than what the manufacturer suggests. "Melanie, the nutritionist, was telling me that a serving of pasta is one-third to half a cup," says Susie, a HAPPY Heart participant: "I'm Italian. We wouldn't even boil water for a quarter cup of pasta. I could easily eat half a pound: that's how we grew up."

Instead of relying on childhood memories, the best way to figure out serving sizes is to pull out your measuring cup and see exactly what two-thirds of a cup of granola looks like poured into the bowl you usually use for cereal. Once you get the hang of it, you can eyeball your servings or use these estimates from the USDA:

- 2 tablespoons of salad dressing: a ping-pong ball
- 3 ounces of cooked meat, fish, or poultry: a deck of cards or the palm of a hand
- 1 ounce of cheese: a pair of dice
- 1 cup of ice cream: a tennis ball
- ¹/₂ cup of cooked rice or pasta: a cupcake wrapper full
- 1 cup of cereal: a tennis ball or fist

Once you're comfortable with various serving sizes, you can then work toward a portion size that is right for you.

Reading a Label

When you read a label, here are some healthy guidelines to follow:

1. Check serving size first, then look at calories.
2. Check fat:
   - Frame of reference: 5 g = 1 tsp/pat of butter
   - Best: less than 5 percent
   - Acceptable: around 10 percent
   - Really high: more than 20 percent
   - Saturated fat: less than 5 percent of daily value
   - No trans fats
3. Check fiber:
   - Good: more than 3 g per serving
   - Excellent: more than 5 g per serving
4. Check sugar:
   - Frame of reference: 5 g = 1 tsp or packet of sugar

- Less than 10 g per serving

5. Check sodium:

- Best: less than 5 percent of daily value
- Acceptable: around 10 percent
- High: more than 20 percent
- Aim for less than 1,500 mg/day total

Eat Breakfast

As Laurie knows, eating breakfast is integral to your overall health. Skipping breakfast has been scientifically proven over the last decade to be associated with skipping fruits and vegetables later in the day, increased calorie intake, decreased physical activity, an increase in your body's insulin response—which can translate into increased fat storage and weight gain—and, not surprisingly, given all those factors, a higher risk of being obese.[10]

British researchers analyzed four studies that looked at the link between breakfast (specifically, eating breakfast cereal) and body weight. Looking at the results for over forty-three thousand people, the analysis found that people, both adults and children, who eat breakfast regularly have a lower BMI and significantly lower waist-hip ratio than those who rarely eat breakfast. "Breakfast really is the most important meal of the day," the study concludes.[11]

Even though that study focused on cereal, there are no hard and fast rules about what breakfast has to look like. Pearsall often recommends that her busy clients think outside the breakfast "box." "I often suggest that they eat a cheese and tomato sandwich for breakfast or have an egg and piece of whole grain toast spread with avocado or some homemade soup," she says. "Eat what you like as long as it's healthy."

Don't Eat and Multitask

Yes, you can read a blog, talk to your husband, and eat a sandwich all at the same time, but that doesn't mean you should. Your mind won't register that sandwich in the same way if you had concentrated solely on it. Scientists at the University of Bristol in England gave twenty-two men and women the same lunch. They asked half to focus on the meal exclusively, while the other half were asked to play solitaire on the computer; both groups were told to finish the whole meal, which was nine small portions of food that ranged from carrots to potato chips. When polled, the group in front of the screen said their lunch was substantially less filling than the crowd who simply ate. An hour later, both groups were told to eat as much dessert as they wanted, and the game players ate twice as many cookies as the mindful eaters.[12]

"It's really important to be engaged with your food and how you eat," says Pearsall. "When you're eating in the car or in front of a screen, you're not really tasting the food." Do your best to eat a meal at a table with minimal distractions. "Turn off the television in the kitchen," she says. "Not only is it simply distracting you from your meal, if you have the news on and something upsetting comes on, it may prompt you to eat more."

Try Not to Drink Your Calories

"Liquid calories, like those from soda, fancy coffee drinks, and juice, are subversive," says Pearsall. "Your body doesn't register them as food because they are not filling physically, yet they often are as caloric as food." To wit: if you drink a sixteen-ounce bottle of Coke, you don't feel satisfied or full, yet you just drank about two hundred calories, which is 10 percent of a two-thousand-calorie daily diet. What's more, if you drink liquid calories when you're actually just thirsty for water, you may be confusing your body even further. "You're giving it the equivalent of food when it didn't ask for it," she explains.

Although kicking the soda habit sounds hard, Christie, a member of HAPPY Heart and former Coke drinker, can tell you otherwise. "I would drink I don't know how many sodas a day," she says, "but I decided to stop, and I found that I acquired a different taste. I don't like them much now." She only drinks them when she eats pizza, which is a great strategy: save your drinks for mealtimes, when you'll be eating solid food and, as such, won't drink as much.

Diet soda isn't a great choice either. One study, published in *Circulation* in 2008, looked at the dietary habits of over 9,500 people ages forty-five to sixty-four and linked diet soda, meat, and fried food consumption to the risk of metabolic syndrome (discussed on page 63).[13] While diet soda may not pack on the calories, the craving for a sweet beverage at a low calorie cost may mislead you into thinking that you can make up for those "lost calories" by indulging in another calorie-laden snack.

Use Your Kitchen

So many of my patients use one kitchen appliance 90 percent of the time: the microwave. If you put some thought and a little—emphasis on little—effort into preparing meals at home, your health will be amply rewarded. The benefits of firing up your own stove or oven are plenty: the cost is a fraction of eating out; you can control your portion size; you can see how much fat and salt goes into a recipe; you can freeze leftovers for future meals or eat them for lunch the next day.

One incentive I suggest to my patients who eat out often is to save all the receipts from food not prepared at home for a month. This includes coffee stops, snacks, and all meals. Then total them up. The following month, do the same thing, but consciously try to cut down (again, small steps: don't stop, just reduce). Total them up again and put the money you saved aside. Continue to downsize until you have enough money for a new kitchen accessory: a steamer, a slow cooker— I just dusted mine off, and can make a great meal for a family of five for less than ten dollars—or a subscription to a cooking magazine like *Cooking Light*. "Cookbooks often just sit on shelves," says Pearsall, "but if you're getting a magazine every month, you're more likely to try the recipes."

If you're unsure of your cooking skills, recruit a friend to go with you to a cooking class or ask your friend to help you in your own kitchen. Here's another option: there are a bunch of cooking-class videos on YouTube, so you can watch, pause, and take notes as necessary.

Grocery-Shop with a Plan

"The biggest thing that influences how you eat at home is how you grocery-shop," says Pearsall. "You can't fill your house with ice cream and chips and then be frustrated with the fact that you're tempted and eat poorly and feel like you have no control."

Here are a few things Pearsall recommends:

1. Before you go shopping, sit down and make a list of every-thing you'll need for the coming week. Don't just think about dinner. What will you have for breakfast? If you're bringing lunch to your work (a good choice, by the way), what will you eat? Will you have enough leftovers from the previous din-ner for lunch or will you need to create a new meal? A little

effort on the front end will save you from overeating on the back end.

2. Only go to the grocery store once a week. "If you have to stop and pick up milk on a Wednesday night and you had a stressful day at work, you're likely to also grab Doritos off the end of an aisle," says Pearsall. If you've got all your supplies at home, there's no chance for impulse purchases.

3. If you have a tough time sticking to your (healthy) list, consider online shopping with delivery. Many grocery stores have this option, and sitting at your computer while you click off your list doesn't carry the same temptations as rolling down the cookie aisle at the store does.

4. If possible, don't bring the kids (or grandkids) with you. "Kids are bad shoppers," says Pearsall with a laugh, "and grocery stores know it." Fruit Loops and Oreos are at eye-level to appeal to the pint-sized crowd. If not bringing them isn't an option, enlist them as helpers: have them cross items off your list, weigh produce, or read labels.

5. Shop after you've had a balanced meal. If you go when your stomach is growling, your body will want foods that are rich in carbs, sugar, and fat. "That's just basic physiology," says Pearsall. "If your body—not your brain—is filling your cart, it'll be full of Cheez-Its and cookies."

6. Shop the perimeter of the store before hitting the middle of it. If you stock up on fruits, veggies, meat, and dairy before you hit the pasta and soda aisles, your cart will already be pretty full. "You'll be more picky about what you put in your cart," she explains.

7. Try not to buy in bulk. "You buy five pounds of pretzels, and you can keep eating them and hardly make a dent," she says. "With a small bag of pretzels, you're much more aware of how

much you've eaten." If you bulk up to save money, portion out the foods ahead of time based on the serving size on the package so you're not tempted to overeat.

8. It's worth repeating one more time: stick to your list. Don't buy a pack of Mint Milano cookies because they are on sale and you'll have them around when company comes over; they'll likely be gone before you have a chance to serve them to somebody besides your family. It's not likely you're going to save those ice cream sandwiches for the grandchildren when they visit next weekend. "If you're going to buy the food, you're going to eat it," says Pearsall, putting it in the simplest—and most honest—terms possible.

Don't Put Any Food Off-Limits

If you say you're never going to eat a cupcake, your favorite dessert, again for the rest of your life, guess what? Images of mini-cakes piled with whipped frosting are going to barrage you until you can't think about anything else. "The foods that hang around in your head are the ones you shouldn't have in your house," Donna Slicis says. "But that doesn't mean you can't have them." Instead, if you're craving a cupcake, tell yourself you can buy one cupcake and enjoy it. Sit down, savor it, relish it, eat it as slowly as you can. Then be done with it. "One cupcake will satisfy you and taste good," says Slicis. "Three or six make you feel nauseous." Pearsall suggests that if you're going to eat food that tempts you, do so when you are out of the house; order it when you are out to eat, or make a special trip to the bakery or store just for it.

But Do Put Limits on Your Eating Times

Because people have various schedules and dinner times, Pearsall isn't a fan of putting a blanket don't-eat-after-8-p.m. rule out there. But she does recommend the idea of closing down the kitchen at a time that's appropriate for your life. "You're most prone to overeat at night," she says, adding that your goal is to wake up feeling hungry. "If your stomach is growling in the morning, that's a good sign," she says. Paige, a member of the HAPPY Heart program, moved her dinner up to 5:30 or 6:00, and doesn't find herself snacking in front of the television, like she used to. "I eat a pear or a piece of fruit if I'm hungry," she says. "I'm much more conscious of the times and foods I eat." The result? She lost ten pounds over two years—and has kept it off.

Just Say No to Diets

I can't point to one patient who went on a restrictive diet, then returned to "regular" eating and was able to maintain the weight she lost. This may sound harsh, but a person who constantly diets shows me she can't manage how she eats. In my mind, chronic dieting actually is a risk factor for obesity.

Not only does the weight not stay off when you unrealistically restrict your calories or eating—the continual weight losses and gains actually harm your body. A study conducted at Seattle's Fred Hutchinson Cancer Research Center concluded that women with more than five major weight losses and gains had about a third less natural killer cell activity—a measurement of a person's immune function that is linked to cancer risk and heart disease—than women who had maintained the same weight for five or more years, even if the steady women were classified as overweight.[14]

If you do have weight to lose, modify your diet with the small steps mentioned above, and aim to reduce your calories by five hundred to one thousand daily. A healthy weight loss is one or two pounds a week, or about 10 percent of your body weight over six months.

Keep a Food Log

If you write down every handful of jelly beans you grab off your coworker's desk, every row of Ritz crackers you eat while watching television, and every item you have for a meal, several studies show that you're more likely to eat less. "Keeping food records was a better predictor of weight loss than were baseline body mass index, exercise, and age," conclude the authors of a groundbreaking study that was published in the *Journal of the American Dietetic Association*. "Monthly as well as cumulative weight loss was directly related to the number of days in which food records were kept."[15] Christie knows this well. "I have a problem with grazing," she says, "and when I write down everything I have eaten, it puts it in a different perspective. Suddenly, I'm thinking, 'Do I really need that bag of chips right now?'"

Even though tracking your eating through the day can be hugely beneficial, Pearsall admits a food log isn't the easiest thing to do in a day already jam-packed with to-do lists. Still, it's clearly worth your effort. Her biggest recommendation is to keep it as simple as possible. Get a small notebook, something that you can tuck into a purse or pocket, or track it on your computer or mobile device. Christie keeps it right in her kitchen. Without changing your eating habits, write down what you ate, when you ate it, and any special circumstances surrounding the situation (for instance: at a dinner with friends; a long day at work; didn't sleep much last night). Write down everything in real time: right after you eat it, log it. If you wait until you're going to bed and try to recall everything you ate that day, "you'll have selective memory," says Pearsall.

Once you have a week of food intake, sit down and dissect the log yourself. Are you overeating at night? Do you regularly reach for sugar in the mid-afternoon? Are you missing breakfast often? You will become your own expert on your individual eating habits. If you can afford it, schedule an hour with a registered dietician who can give you additional insight into your eating habits. (Find one in your area at eatright.org.)

The Skinny on Supplements

There's a joke often told at medical conferences when the subjects of vitamins and supplements come up: America has the healthiest sewer system in the world. Implied, of course, is that the vitamins people take aren't being put to good use in their bodies, but rather they are being flushed down the drain with their urine. Kind of funny, but supplements aren't really a joke.

It's perplexing to me that billions of dollars are spent annually on dietary substances that have not been scientifically proven to be beneficial. While some people take recommended supplements to complement traditional medical treatment for conditions such as high blood pressure, high cholesterol, or heart disease, many other people take supplements because they believe that "natural" substances are less harmful and equally effective. In one study, I looked at patterns of *complementary and alternative medicine* (CAM) use by patients with cardiovascular disease and found that 68 percent were using some form of CAM. The most commonly used therapies included vitamins and nutritional supplements.[16] Many of the patients were on supplements that could have potentially interacted with the heart medications, and, what's more troubling, the majority of patients did not share this information with their physician. An example is red yeast rice. While it may lower cholesterol, it is very similar to statins and may result in many of the side effects, including liver issues, and drug interactions noted with statins.

If you are going to spend money on a supplement, be an educated consumer and communicate with your doctor. She should know about everything you're taking, so she can be vigilant about tests, drug interactions, and side effects.

Here are the supplements with scientific data behind them that I recommend to my patients if they're interested.

SUPPLEMENT	THE SCIENCE?	RDA	BEST SOURCES
Flaxseed*	• Whole flaxseed may reduce cholesterol levels, but current data is not compelling. • There is no evidence for flaxseed oil.	• There are no specific guidelines for flaxseed, but there are for omega-3 fatty acids: 1 g daily. • A tablespoon of ground flaxseed contains about 1.8 g of omega-3s.	• Flaxseeds • Supplements
Fish oil*	• Reduces risk of death from heart arrhythmia. • Has a possible anti-inflammatory effect. • Is helpful in lowering triglycerides at higher doses.	• 3.5 oz. of oily fish is recommended, twice a week, or 1 g fish oil (omega-3 fatty acid) per day. • Larger doses (2 to 4 g) are required to lower triglycerides.	• Oily fish (salmon, trout, mackerel, herring, sardines, among others) • Supplements

* Note: Both fish and flaxseed oil contain omega-3s, so you should choose one or the other, not both.

SUPPLEMENT	THE SCIENCE?	RDA	BEST SOURCES
Folic acid	• Aids in the creation of red blood cells. • Reduces the risk of neural tube defects in the fetus immediately prior to and during pregnancy. • Is not recommended to prevent heart disease, except in cases of elevated homocysteine levels.	• 400 micrograms (µg)/day for everybody • 600 µg during pregnancy • 500 µg while nursing • 1 mg for elevated homocysteine levels	• Fortified cereals (check the label) • Spinach (¹/₂ cup has 100 g) • Rice (¹/₂ cup has 65 g) • Supplements
Vitamin C	• Although eating a diet rich in vitamin-C-dense fruits and vegetables appears to reduce risk of cancer and heart disease, straight supplements have not been shown to provide similar benefits. • Limits the production of free radicals (negative molecules that disrupt cells and can lead to heart disease and cancer). • Promotes the healing of wounds.	• 75 mg • 120 mg if breast-feeding	• Broccoli • Bell peppers • Kale • Cauliflower • Strawberries • Citrus fruits
Vitamin E	• Not recommended to specifically prevent cardiovascular disease, although it limits the production of free radicals.	• 15 mg	• Sunflower oil • Almonds • Safflower oil • Peanut butter • Supplements

SUPPLEMENT	THE SCIENCE?	RDA	BEST SOURCES
Vitamin D	Reduces risk of • Osteoporosis • Hip fracture • Cardiovascular-related death.	• 600 international units (IU) • >70 years of age 800 IU • Although needs may vary, your physician may want to check the level of vitamin D in your blood.	• Dairy products • Sunshine • Supplements
Calcium	• Reduces risk of osteoporosis, hip fracture. • Has minimal effect on cardiovascular risk. • Limited data suggests possible increased risk of heart attack.	• 1,000 to 1,200 mg • 1,300 mg if pregnant	• Milk • Yogurt • Cheese • Cabbage • Kale • Broccoli • Calcium supplements if necessary

Three Easy First Steps Across the Nutrition Bridge

1. **Clean house.** Go through the cupboards and get rid of foods that were purchased on a whim or that are unhealthy and contain empty calories; you can't mindlessly eat what you don't have in the house. While the kids may complain at first when the box of Oreos disappears, a whole-grain nutrition bar or bag of carrots and celery may work just as well.

2. **Stay grounded.** If you're contemplating eating or buying a new food, ask yourself, How many steps did this food go through from coming out of the ground until it hit the shelves at the store? If the answer is more than three, pass it up.

3. **Keep it moving.** Fiber doesn't just do your GI system good; it can also help prevent heart disease, according to a study published in 2011 and conducted at Northwestern University in Chicago. "Younger (twenty to thirty-nine years) and middle-aged (forty to fifty-nine years) adults with the highest fiber intake, compared to those with the lowest fiber intake, showed a statistically significant lower lifetime risk for cardiovascular disease," said Hongyan Ning, MD, lead author. Aim for 25 g a day or more, ideally from whole foods, not processed supplements or drinks.[17]

chapter seven

The Relationship Bridge

Madeline had a family that would send Dear Abby running for the hills. Her closest family relationships—those with her mother, her ex-husband, and her daughter—were totally draining her. Her mother, who had previously broken her back, was prone to blacking out. "I called her every hour of every day," said Madeline, the one of six siblings who stepped up to be her mother's main caretaker, "and if she didn't answer the phone, I'd jump in my car and go to her house to check on her."

In addition to being on watch 24/7, Madeline often felt guilted into accompanying her mother to lunch in a restaurant, where she preferred to eat daily. "I hate eating out," Madeline says, "but I did it because that's what she wanted." Her ex-husband, who cheated on her multiple times, still wanted to be her best friend. "He was calling me all the time, telling me about his relationship problems," she says. On top of all that, her daughter tried to commit suicide multiple times. "I was off the wall," she admits. "At one point, I just gave up answering the phone when she would call. I just couldn't deal with it anymore. I realize how selfish that sounds, but I just couldn't deal."

The HAPPY Heart group, which bonded faster than superglue, gave Madeline insight into the kind of relationships she lacked—and desperately needed—in her life: namely, supportive friendships that energize you and make you feel happy and whole, not ones that zap your energy and leave you frustrated and hostile. With the encouragement of the HAPPY Heart group, she was able to take a step back and realize how much she gave to those three relationships and how little she got in return. She didn't eliminate those relationships from her life (well, she did tell her ex that he couldn't call her anymore), but she did put them in perspective. And that perspective, for the first time in her life, included her own feelings and needs.

Madeline finally realized that she had done all she could for her daughter, and, although she would always love and support her, she couldn't handle the drama anymore. "I told her, 'You're forty-two years old. You made your life. I can't take care of you anymore.'" She remembers, "I wouldn't have had the confidence to tell her that without the support of my HAPPY Heart girls." Her phone calls to her mother have decreased to three times a day, and instead of spending endless hours lunching in restaurants, where Madeline often can't find heart-healthy options, they now do errands together or meet for coffee occasionally. "I've learned to pull back from her a little because my friends kept telling me you can't be your mother's keeper forever," she says. "I always was."

She even takes her new I-deserve-respect attitude to relationships that aren't as troublesome. "When my other daughter, who is a little hyper, gets angry about something when we're talking on the phone, I just hold the phone away from my ear until she calms down," she says, "and if she doesn't, I simply tell her, 'I will call you back when I am ready.'"

While you might not have as complicated a family situation as Madeline's, chances are, the relationships in your life have challenged you at some point. Relationships, whether they're with friends, parents, siblings, children, or a partner, make up the bulk of our lives and, as such, are bound to hit some speed bumps along the way. The connections we make as we go through life allow us to grow, learn, share, and love. They bring us our greatest happiness and our most profound grief. The best relationships are like a fine wine; they become more interesting and fulfilling over time. At their best, they can fill you with euphoria. At their worst, unhealthy relationships carry the opposite effect; feelings like guilt, resentment, hostility, and frustration can take their toll on your health.

Having healthy, meaningful relationships is just as important to your well-being as being at a healthy weight and not smoking; in fact, research shows that the relationship advantage is about the same as the mortality difference between smokers and nonsmokers. Health coach Donna Slicis tells a story about how a HAPPY Heart participant was mediating a fight between her son and his girlfriend, as she was prone to do. Realizing how unhealthy the bickering was both for her to be around and the couple to be doing, she finally just left, midfight. "She said, 'This isn't good for me. I have somewhere I belong,'" recounts Slicis, adding that the weekly HAPPY Heart meeting was starting soon, which is where she needed to be. "We can't scientifically measure situations and responses like that, but we know how important they are. You find a few women you like, and you end up loving them. And you blossom in response."

The study of relationships and their outcome on your health is fairly new, but the outcomes of the research all point definitively in one direction: both the quality and quantity of your relationships matter. In 2010, researchers at Brigham Young University and the University of North Carolina at Chapel Hill pooled 148 studies that involved relationships and health. Looking at the results from more than 300,000 men and women, they concluded that those with higher levels of social interaction were, on average, 50 percent more likely to be alive than those with poor social connections in the study's follow-up period (an average of seven-and-a-half years). The results were very egalitarian; both men and women of all ages and in various states of health were all shown to benefit from friendly relationships.[1]

A similar study is one of my favorites and reinforces everything I try to emphasize with my patients, HAPPY Hearters, friends, and family. In a nutshell, a 2008 study from the University of California at San Diego found that happiness is contagious. Looking at data from over 4,700 people over two decades, researchers found that if you have a friend who lives within a mile and is generally happy, you're about 25 percent more likely to be happy yourself; spouses, nearby siblings, and next-door neighbors have similar effects.[2] I love this study because it proves that your happiness depends on the happiness of others with whom you are connected, and it empowers you with the knowledge that you can help your close relationships by being happy. In addition, it provides further justification for seeing happiness, like health, as a collective phenomenon.

The HAPPY Heart group is just one example of a supportive social community; you can find them in your neighborhood, in your church, at work, at the gym, through groups devoted to a hobby, either online or in person, and of course, through a web of friends from different places and times in your life. Chances are, you are more likely to find similarly minded positive people at a spin class or a reading group, rather than sitting on bar stools, drowning their sorrows. Like all things worth keeping in your life, you need to consciously maintain your relationships; you can't put a relationship on autopilot and expect it to sustain itself. Nurturing and engaging in the relationships that bring you love and warmth—and, alternatively, cutting off or minimizing the ones that are unhealthy—is well worth the effort, both for your mind and body. When you have a strong social network, you can actually enhance your health.

I'll go through the research for three topics that relate intimately to relationships—loneliness, friendships, and marriage—then talk about how you can create or sustain a robust, healthy social network.

Loneliness

One is the loneliest—and perhaps unhealthiest—number. Feeling alone in the world can have a detrimental effect on your health and heart as the broken heart syndrome (discussed on page 19) illustrates. The death of a spouse; a move across the country; a divorce that alienates you from your former friends; a new, all-consuming job: all of these situations can elicit feelings of isolation and desperation. To be clear, spending time alone isn't a bad thing; we all need solitary time to decompress and rejuvenate our minds and spirits. But feeling isolated, even when you're surrounded by people, is the kind of lonely I'm talking about.

Part of my connection to women in need arose from my move to Nova Scotia, when my children were little and my husband at the time was working long hours on his fellowship. I had gone from working in a thriving practice and being surrounded by friends to finding myself alone with small children, living in a new country, and not working for a few months. I felt the physical toll this took on me. After a few months, I found women with whom I connected through a running group and through our church, and I felt back to normal. Those first few months were very tough for me, though. While I wasn't entirely alone, I lacked the social connections that had previously been a very important part of my life.

"Loneliness is the discrepancy between your achieved and desired level of social contact, and that has important implications," commented Chris Segrin, PhD, a behavioral scientist and head of the department of communication at the University of Arizona. "The portrait of a lonely person is very difficult to paint because what is really important is what is in your head."[3]

When you feel lonely, that perception ricochets through your whole body.

Loneliness Affects the Cardiovascular System

Andrew Steptoe, along with some colleagues at the University College London, looked at the body's response to loneliness in 240 people, aged forty-seven to fifty-nine. Lonely women were particularly susceptible to higher blood pressure, and lonely individuals had greater levels of *fibrogen*, a protein in the blood that can lead to increased blood clotting, decreased activity of natural *killer cells* (blood cells that fight infection), and higher levels of cortisol, the stress-related hormone that predisposes you to dangerous abdominal fat.[4] The high blood pressure findings were investigated further in a 2010 study out of the University of Chicago, which looked at the four-year cumulative effect on blood pressure in lonely people. "Loneliness at the outset of the study predicted increases in systolic blood pressure in years two, three, and four," commented the authors, noting that the effect was independent of perceived stress, depressive symptoms, social support, and other seemingly related symptoms.[5]

Loneliness Can Make You More Predisposed to Illness

In 2011, Steve Cole, PhD, a professor of medicine at UCLA who studies the genetic roots of loneliness, looked at the number of pro-inflammatory immune cells in adults who are lonely and who are not. These cells, which are one of the first things that get activated when the body is injured and can, if not quieted, lead to cardiovascular disease, were at abnormally high levels in the bodies of the lonely adults.[6] Additional experiments from Cole had similar results: he has repeatedly found that loneliness is linked to harmful inflammation and a decrease in helpful antibody production and antiviral activity. "We found that what counts at the level of gene expression is not how many people you know, it's how many you feel really close to over time," Cole told *Science Daily* about his research.[7]

Loneliness Discourages a Healthy Lifestyle

In 2010, Segrin surveyed 265 adults, ages nineteen to eighty-five, and found that those who reported that they were lonely, in comparison to those who were not lonely, did not get adequate sleep (or feel fresh and rejuvenated after sleeping); did not enjoy leisure activities, like swimming; were not able to manage stress effectively; and did not take medicines as prescribed. Loneliness, like depression, is a condition that predisposes you not to take care of yourself properly. Lonely adults tend to consume more alcohol, eat foods higher in fat, and get less exercise than their more social peers.[8]

Friendships

When people think of a social network, the first thing that comes to mind is friendships. The importance of friendships has been substantially documented; people with strong social relationships are more likely to live longer; be less susceptible to cognitive decline with aging (those endless games of bridge keep your mind active!); be more resistant to infectious disease; and have a better prognosis when it comes to life-threatening illnesses. Current research has focused more on the quality of the relationships: how friends influence one another and how the depth of friendships may be more important than the number of friends one has. Some new interesting studies and their findings include the following.

Friends Can Point Your Lifestyle Needle in the Healthy Direction

For two years, Shiriki K. Kumanyika, PhD, MPH, and her colleagues at the University of Pennsylvania School of Medicine in Philadelphia conducted an exercise-based trial on 344 African-American adults, a group particularly at risk for obesity and cardiovascular complications. The group was divided into three categories: people who exercised alone; pairs who were both given high support; and pairs, where one person was given low support. The goal over the two years was to maintain a 5 to 10 percent weight loss, and they would be monitored at six, twelve, eighteen, and twenty-four months. At the end of two years, all main participants had lost, on average, 5.3 pounds. But those with gung-ho partners were more likely to succeed; they found that if a partner lost at least 5 percent of their body weight, the other partner was more inclined to have similar success.[9]

Anecdotally, I've found a workout buddy to be one of the most important factors determining success in an exercise program. The HAPPY Heart participants love the group walks, tai chi classes, yoga classes . . . anything that involves their friends and occasional chatter and laughter. Having a friend by your side as you physically challenge yourself just makes it intrinsically feel easier.

Friends Can Also Influence Poor Lifestyle Choices

HAPPY Heart wellness coach Susan Lane, who teaches smoking cessation classes, finds that smokers who have the hardest time quitting are those who are always around smokers. Her experience was confirmed when, in 2010, researchers at MGH studied data involving alcohol consumption and social networks. They found that a person's network—namely, their relatives and friends—significantly influenced the amount of alcohol they consumed. People were 50 percent more likely to drink heavily if a person they were connected to did so; the percentage dropped to 36 percent for two degrees of separation (like a friend of a friend), and 15 percent for three degrees. In addition, intense relationships, like a marriage, had a greater effect. Heavy drinking by a wife increased the husband's likelihood of drinking heavily by 196 percent, while heavy drinking by a husband increased a wife's chances for drinking heavily by 126 percent.

On the other hand, if a direct contact abstained, a person was 29 percent more likely to abstain as well. At two degrees of separation it was 21 percent, and at three, 5 percent. What's more, each additional abstainer in a person's life reduced the chance that she would drink heavily by 10 percent. (A person's neighbors and coworkers didn't have the same effect.[10])

A similar effect on body mass index was proven in a study that used data from the Framingham Heart Study, a comprehensive, multi-generational study that focuses on cardiovascular disease and was published in the *New England Journal of Medicine.* Researchers found that if your sibling or spouse becomes obese, your chances of becoming obese go up by about 40 percent. If a person you consider to be a friend becomes obese, your chance of mimicking your friend's habits increases by 57 percent. And, most astonishingly of all, if one person in a set of mutual friends—you both hold each other in high regard—raises her BMI into the unhealthy range, the other has a 171 percent chance of doing so herself.[11]

The relationship seems to stretch out to three degrees, and the connection is so strong, the researchers call obesity *contagious.* "Weight gain could spread through a variety of social ties from person to person, but they had to be close relationships," write Nicholas A. Christakis, MD, MPH, PhD, a professor at Harvard Medical School, and James H. Fowler, PhD, a professor at University of California in San Diego, in *Connected: The Surprising Power of Our Social Networks and How They Shape Our Lives.* "You may not know him personally, but your friend's husband's coworker can make you fat, and your sister's friend's boyfriend can make you thin." It is important to note that the relationship seems to work in both directions: both for gaining and losing weight.[12]

Christakis continued his research in another study, looking at the effects of health traits on friendship ties. Using the same data, he looked carefully at the role of social engagement and relationships on health behavior. In this study, he found that both BMI and smoking influence one's choice of which new friends are chosen and existing friendships are dissolved. "The fact that homophily [love of the same] is evident for . . . BMI and smoking traits but that only weak evidence is present for the other traits [which include blood pressure, depression, birth order, and personality type] suggests that, in general, people seek out individuals who have come to resemble them or dissolve ties with those who come not to resemble them in obvious, health-related ways," he writes in the conclusion.[13]

In a final note, Christakis and Fowler are starting to investigate the genetic roots of our friendships. Preliminary research, published in early 2011, found a connection between a person's social network and the DRD2 gene, which is associated with a propensity for alcoholism; there is a possibility that friends share the same genetic clusters.[14] While the study is far from conclusive, it points to the importance of the next frontier: considering the health implications of one's friends.

The Quality of the Friendship Matters, Especially When You're Feeling Stressed

Looking at how ambivalence, often described as a state of mixed feelings, influenced cardiovascular functioning, researchers at Brigham Young University had 107 people, both males and females, talk about positive and negative life events. Accompanying each participant was either a supportive or an ambivalent same-sex friend. The biggest changes in blood pressure were recorded when somebody was talking about a negative event with an ambivalent friend nearby; in addition, those who brought ambivalent friends had higher resting heart rate levels than those who had supportive friends. The experts concluded that individuals may not be able to fully relax in the company of ambivalent friends and may not benefit from their support during stressful times.[15] A study conducted at the University of Utah found similar results: looking at the positive aspects of relationships, researchers found that the positive relationships were most beneficial to blood pressure.[16]

Assess Your Relationships

I often recommend to my patients that an easy way to assess their relationships is to think of their interactions with another person on a numeric scale, with 1 being totally unhealthy (being with that person usually brings up feelings of fear, anger, and resentment) and 10 being very healthy (being together brings up feelings of happiness and fulfillment). If most of your interactions in one relationship are clustered around a seven or greater, then it's likely that's a consistent, healthy relationship. If the numbers swing from two to nine to three, the relationship is likely tempestuous and volatile and will need some TLC: quality time together (or with a therapist) where you decide to make changes so that the relationship can level out. Finally, anything consistently below a five is probably a relationship you're better off without.

Marriage

Science has shown that the benefits of a good marriage are multiple and wide-ranging. While similar benefits may exist for unmarried, long-term domestic partnerships, these partnerships have not been extensively studied so direct parallels cannot be assumed. When you're married, your spouse presumably has your back. A spouse might notice when your mood or body is out of whack, can be a sounding board for your health questions, and is your advocate in appropriate medical situations.

Before you read further, though, I want you to know that whether or not you have a partner in life, your life can be fulfilling and healthy.

Your social network, which can easily be defined as close friends and family members, can help provide the support that those in a long-term relationship receive from a partner. Remember that it is always better to be alone than to be in a relationship that compromises your health, safety, or core values.

In 2007, the U.S. Department of Health and Human Services summarized the research that had been done to that point on the effects of marriage on health. "Married people are generally healthier than unmarried people," the paper begins, before diving into the research.[17] Following are their findings as well as some other interesting studies about marriage and health.

Lifestyle Choices Are Influenced by Marriage in Both Positive and Negative Ways

Married people are less likely to both consume alcohol and drink heavily, but studies show mixed results with regard to smoking. In addition, weight gain, usually an amount less than five pounds, is associated with marriage, and evidence suggests that men are more likely to be more sedentary once they get married.[18]

Marriage Does a Heart Good

Both married men and women have lower chances of suffering a heart attack, and if they do, have improved odds of getting better than their unmarried counterparts. In fact, at a cardiac rehab program at MGH, 92 percent of the people who dropped out were single, divorced, widowed, or separated; it takes a fair bit of encouragement to stick with cardiac rehabilitation, and significant others can provide the support that is often necessary for success.

For women over fifty, the risk of cardiovascular disease goes up 60 percent for divorced women and 30 percent for widowed women as compared to women who are still married. "Emotional distress and socioeconomic status account for the higher risk of cardiovascular disease among divorced women," conclude the authors of a study, published in the *Journal of Marriage and Family*.[19] For the majority of women, divorce is a highly traumatic event and is perceived as a sign of failure. Many women and men grieve this loss alone—and, in some cases, for the rest of their lives. If you're contemplating or undergoing a divorce, or have gone through one, please don't be shy: reach out to friends who might not realize you're hurting as much as you are. If that feels too overwhelming, mentally flip the tables: if your friend were grieving, wouldn't you want to help her?

Mental Health Is Helped Through Marriage

Marriage reduces depressive symptoms for both men and women, although getting divorced increases them. Divorce is obviously a stressful time, but getting divorced does not condemn one to depression. Try to approach the situation as a challenge; do your best to navigate the divorce while maintaining both your dignity and a respectful relationship with your ex.

Marriage Increases Your Life Span

A 2006 paper published in the *Journal of Epidemiology and Community Health* found that, over an eight-year period, people who never married were 58 percent more likely to die during that period than those who were married.[20]

Even When Marriage Ends, It Still Affects Your Health

The benefits of marriage are so substantial that when you lose a spouse, either to death or divorce, your health takes a serious dive and may not fully recover. In a 2009 study, published in the *Journal of Health and Social Behavior*, researchers looked at the marital and health histories of nine thousand men and women in their fifties and sixties. When somebody lost a spouse, an individual was prone to have 20 percent more chronic health issues and 23 percent more "limitations" that affected using the stairs and walking longer distances.[21] Remarriage mitigated some of the symptoms but did not bring the once-single person's health back to the level they were at in the first marriage. "We argue that losing a marriage through divorce or widowhood is extremely stressful and that a high-stress period takes a toll on health," commented researcher Linda J. Waite, a professor of sociology at the University of Chicago.[22] Please note that the message here is not that divorce or widowhood condemns you to a less healthy life. Rather, it just means that you need to make your health a priority and to work harder to get back the health benefits that you previously enjoyed.

Clearly, a happy marriage is like a great health insurance policy: it has you covered. But what about an unhappy one? Current research is adding a more helpful layer to the previous all-is-good research; looking at the nature of the relationship, it's clear that a respectful, supportive, and loving marriage is the most beneficial kind. Scientists are discovering that the most important thing is not if there's a wedding ring, but how partners treat each other.

A Hostile Marriage Can Seriously Impact Your Immune System

At Ohio State University, researchers inflicted small wounds on forty-two otherwise healthy married couples, whose ages ranged from twenty-two to seventy-seven, and did two experiments. In the first one, one partner was asked to talk about an aspect of themselves they wanted to change, and the other partner was asked to encourage them in a positive way. In the second one, which happened a few months later, each partner was asked to bring up a divisive issue, like financial matters. The wounds healed accordingly. After the first session, most people were healed after five days; after the second session, it took them six days. But in couples that were hostile toward each other, the healing times were six and seven days, respectively.[23] "This study was carried out on healthy people, and a lot of them were young," commented Patricia Price, director of the Wound Healing Research Unit in Cardiff at the University of Wales College of Medicine, in *New Scientist*. "So imagine the effect on people who are elderly or already immunosuppressed. Some wounds, such as leg ulceration associated with diabetic foot disease, can take months to heal. The implications of stress for these people could be enormous."[24]

A Strained Marriage Can Keep Your Body in a Constantly Stressed State

Led by Timothy W. Smith, PhD, a professor of clinical psychology at the University of Utah who has extensively studied the connection between marriage and health, a group of researchers looked at the effect of marital conflict on cardiovascular health. They found that, compared to the effects of collaborative problem solving, conflict increased blood pressure, cardiac output, and the effect of adrenaline on the heart.[25] Chronic exposure to marital stress, and the accompanying ups and downs of blood pressure and other stress-related responses, may do long-term damage to the cardiovascular system.

Marital Discontent Can Lead to Progression of Heart Artery Disease

Looking at the cardiac health and relationship quality of 154 couples that had been married, on average, for just over thirty-six years, researchers found that relationships low in warmth and high in dominating behaviors lead to increased calcium in the arteries of the heart in women and men.[26] There is a direct correlation between the calcium in the arteries and the risk of developing heart disease.

A Good Marriage Benefits Your Sleep

Researchers at the University of Pittsburgh investigated the link between sleep quality and relationship quality and history. Analyzing data from over 2,100 women, they found that happily married women reported better-quality, continuous sleep and fewer sleep-related complaints than less happily married women.[27] (They also looked at the connection between sleep and stability in a relationship and found that women who had been in one stable relationship for at least eight years had more productive sleep than women who were either consistently single or those who were in multiple relationships.[28]) The association with lasting relationships could be attributed to both physiological causes (hormones like oxytocin that make you calm) and lifestyle contributions (routine schedules, fewer unhealthy habits).

When It Comes to Cardiac Issues, a Healthy Marriage Is Powerful Medicine

In a study published in the *American Journal of Cardiology*, researchers looked at 189 patients with heart failure and interviewed them about their marital quality. They found that, over an eight-year period, marital quality predicted survival, especially when the patient was female. "[It] did so substantially better than [other factors] like psychological distress, hostility, neuroticism, self-efficacy, optimism, and breadth of perceived emotional support," the authors concluded.[29]

Build the Bridge to Better Relationships

Even though relationships may seem intuitive, they're far from it. It takes time, thoughtfulness, and effort to develop friendships and partners who can enhance your life (and vice versa), as well as relationships with family members that are truly fulfilling. Here are some ways to find and foster relationships.

Be Chatty

You never know where a meaningful relationship might begin, so open yourself up to the possibility by simply engaging somebody. A compliment—"I like your hair/shoes/purse"—is an easy way to start, as is a simple, "How's it going?" Based on the response, you'll naturally know if the person is open to a conversation or isn't interested. Similarly, don't let your telephone gather dust. While texting and Facebooking are efficient and often fulfilling ways of communicating, hearing somebody's voice and laughing out loud together (not just LOL-ing from one keyboard to another) connects you in a deeper, different way. I have a friend who calls at least one friend from her past every week. One week, it could be her best friend from fourth grade; the next week it could be her roommate from her single days in New York City.

So often, as women, we are taught to be safe and in trying to become safe, we disengage ourselves from the world. It doesn't have to be this way. Smile, make eye contact, and interact with others at a level that feels comfortable to you.

Get Together

Sounds really basic, but people are always in a rush/get-it-done mode these days. Dinner plans for a Friday night get rescheduled—and eventually cancelled—because you always have to work late; a date for coffee seems so flexible and easy to schedule that it never gets put on the books; a morning walk is postponed because of bad weather, and then life gets in the way. For any relationship to grow, you need to take time to nurture it. (This is especially true of a marriage; date nights, even if that just means a walk in the park while holding hands, are vital to intimate, loving marriages.) While it is always possible to rebuild a relationship, maintaining and nurturing the important relationships in our life—and not letting them dry up on the vine—is the best and healthiest way to go.

One of my friends who is in a happy, long-term marriage and who is a very busy professional (and married to another busy professional) has insisted upon a Saturday night date since the birth of their children. They book a dinner reservation and a sitter, go out and spend their evening catching up on each other's week and reflecting and remembering how much they love one another.

Unearth Your Supportive Community

Make a list of at least three people you could call if you had an emergency; people who would come to your house or bedside as soon as possible and do their best to take care of you. Can't think of three? Then you have some work to do. Supportive communities are buried in the woodwork of our lives; sometimes you just don't know they're there—or you take them for granted. When you go to the gym or to church or when you're out mowing your lawn, take off your blinders and, again, strike up a conversation. You never know what may come of it. If that feels too intimidating, take a class that interests you or volunteer out of your house; the group setting and shared interest will naturally lend themselves to conversation and friendship.

Listen Well and Fight Fairly

Book upon book has been written on how to listen (even if women are from Venus and men are from Mars) and how to avoid hysterical catfights with your spouse. While I invite you to investigate any communication style that you think might work for you, I often distill my rules into three easy ones:

1. **Treat conflict like dirty laundry.** Toss whatever is bugging you out there and discuss the source of conflict. Get it soapy and spin it out—share and discuss your individual feelings about the conflict—and then arrive at a point where it's clean: the problem is either solved, you have agreed to disagree about it, or you realize you need to seek an objective source, like a friend, relative, or professional.

2. **Respect, respect, respect.** Treat your partner as you expect to be treated. Listen to what is being said, even if a work project or a bum knee distracts you.

3. **Be open to criticism.** Sometimes we can see the weaknesses in others with 20/20 vision but need a little help in the self-reflection department. When the mirror is turned back on you, do your best to keep an open mind.

Terminate the Tough Relationships

Many of us find every excuse in the world to procrastinate when it comes to dealing with unhealthy relationships; it's often easier to stay in a holding pattern than to take action. Whether with a spouse or significant other, a friend or a family member, it's important, for your health's sake, for you to step up.

If you find yourself in a relationship that is consistently causing undue stress, the first step is determining the importance of the relationship in your life: is this a relationship you're interested in saving? If so, remember that relationship problems do not occur in a vacuum; likely both parties have contributed to the situation, so examine your own role in creating the stress. In addition, if you want to maintain the relationship, realize that it may require professional advice to get back on track.

Sometimes, however, relationships are beyond repair. In these cases, write down the relationship facts, as objectively and specifically, as you can. Remember all the details surrounding the loss of relationship satisfaction, and put it in a safe place so you can remember it when time has blurred your memories. Remember the initials D-O-I, which stand for "definition of insanity": that's when you do the same thing over and over again, expecting a different outcome. It's understandable to hope that the behavior of another will change (and as such, we're prone to offering second, third, and fourth chances), but the reality is, you can't change anybody except yourself.

When you find yourself longing for the terminated relationship (a very natural feeling, by the way), bring in the support of friends and family who have your best intentions in their heart. Break out the journal entry you wrote and read it. In your head, replace the vision of that person with a vision of you doing something very positive for yourself as a gift for getting out of the unhealthy relationship.

Don't Sweat the Small Stuff

Everybody, including you, has their own little tics: maybe you bite your nails, maybe you interrupt conversations too often, maybe you aren't always top notch with your table manners. Yes, over time, those little personality quirks can get annoying, but do your best to mentally zoom out and remember that you're dealing with a person you like, not a habit you don't.

Warning: I'm going to sound like your mother for a second when I say this, but gossip serves no purpose. At a minimum, it can make you feel bad about yourself ("Did she really say that?"); blown out of proportion, it can create unnecessary drama and severely hurt feelings. To quote my—and probably everybody else's—mother: "If you can't say something nice about someone, don't say anything at all."

But Remember the Small Stuff

Give a boost to any relationship by doing something special for that person. It doesn't have to be huge or expensive: bring a coworker a book you have read and think she might like; take your partner out for a surprise dinner; give your family the gift of a technology-free weekend (turn off the phone and computer, and focus on the people you love in your life).

Parenting Your Parents

I was thirty-nine years old when my mother had a major stroke. I suddenly found myself in the "sandwich generation": both my one-year-old and my mother required full-time care and attention. I lived halfway across the country from my parents, so I immediately flew home to help arrange the details of Mom's care. Suddenly I was interviewing caretakers, just as I had interviewed nannies for my kids. The upside of the situation, if there were such a thing, is that I was very familiar with the nuances of hiring: background checks, negotiating salaries, and arranging hours. Two dear friends and colleagues had experienced a similar situation with their parents, and they were invaluable resources for both advice and support. Another benefit: I realized that eldercare could be just as demanding and time consuming as caring for my young family and I could only be pulled in so many directions. Just as personal experience does with every situation, it made me instantly more empathic to my patients who were in the position of parenting their parents.

Everyone's situation is different, but the common theme is this: do what you can, but don't expect to do it all. Here are some ideas that can help you simultaneously care for both your parents and yourself:

- **Engage the professionals.** An eldercare attorney can help you figure out how to pay for care, while an agency can assist in finding care providers. A geriatric care manager can help with everything from nursing facilities to community resources. If you work outside the home, ask the human resources department about the Family Leave Act.

- **Don't go it alone.** Even if you end up shouldering the bulk of the care, be sure to line up others—siblings, friends, a paid care provider—to give you regular, frequent breaks. When you do get a break, do your best not to instantly start on chores or errands: go for a walk or run; see a movie; have coffee with a friend; or otherwise take care of yourself. And be sure to keep up your health with regular doctor's appointments; mention that you are a caregiver to your doctor, as the additional load can affect your stress levels and health.

- **Remember that your parent is still an adult.** Don't just swoop in and take care of everything. Let her make all appropriate decisions and complete any tasks she is capable of, even if it takes extra time. Doing so lets your parent maintain her dignity and sense of self.

- **Find a support group.** Whether it's a friend or coworker who has gone through a similar situation or a formal group, talking with other people who are going through the same situation can mentally ease your mind and help you realize you're not alone.

- **Realize that people don't change much.** If you had a tough relationship with the parent you are now caring for, chances are it will still be trying, especially because he or she is in poor health. Do your best to remember you can't control how your parent acts, but you can most definitely control how you respond. When things get too intense, walk away if you need to; deflect the conversation; say in a calm, objective tone, "I don't like how you're treating me"; or suggest that the pair of you work on a shared project, like a photo album, to talk about your past in a less confrontational way.

Three Easy First Steps Across the Relationship Bridge

1. **Use a three-question quiz.** Before you say something that might cause hostility or anger, ask yourself: Is it true? Is it kind? Is it helpful? So often we speak without truly thinking through our words; being more diligent with word choice and messages can go a long way in keeping a relationship strong.

2. **Grab somebody's hand and hold on.** While it might feel a little awkward at first, the skin-to-skin contact naturally helps your body relax. A study, published in the journal *Psychological Science*, bears this out. Neuroscientists recruited sixteen married women and put each of them in an MRI machine so they could monitor their brain waves and so they couldn't see when a mild electric shock would touch their ankle. They were each shocked three times: the first time, the woman was alone; the second, she held the hand of a stranger; and the third, she held the hand of her husband. Anticipating the shock, the women's brains were mobilized into action, creating a response similar to how it reacts to stress. But when a woman had a hand to hold, her brain was significantly calmer. Although wives in the happiest marriages showed the biggest change when they held their husbands' hands, the effect of a stranger's hand was also helpful.[30] "We found when you're holding a hand—any hand—the parts of your brain responsible for mobilizing your body into action calm down," said James A. Coan, PhD, assistant professor of psychology at the University of Virginia and the author of the lead study. "It doesn't matter whose hand it is."[31]

   When I was flying home from my father's funeral, the plane encountered a significant technical problem. My daughters were sitting two rows ahead of me and immediately looked back to me for reassurance. I smiled and calmly told them to relax, that everything would be okay. Under my breath I explained to the total stranger sitting next to me that it had been a tough week and that I really could use a hand to hold onto as we initiated emergency landing procedures. He kindly and discretely took my hand and held it tight through the landing, releasing it only when we were safely on the ground. The simple gesture made an enormous difference.

3. **No sudden moves.** Abide by this quote from author Garrison Keillor, which is perfect for both marriage and most other relationships in your life. "The rules for marriage are the same as for a lifeboat," he writes: "No sudden moves, don't crowd the other person, and keep all disastrous thoughts to yourself."[32]

chapter eight

The Communication Bridge

A few years ago, Teri, a forty-eight-year-old woman who lives in Boston, was hit with the diagnosis that one in eight women in America, including me, receives at some point in her life: breast cancer.[1] As the mother of three daughters, ages twelve, fourteen, and eighteen, the thought of not seeing them receive their high school diplomas, not walking down the aisle on their wedding days, or not meeting her grandchildren, had Teri reeling. Her husband, a quiet man who expressed his love for her through hard work, not words, had a hard time discussing the situation at length. She knew he would support and care for her, but she also knew he didn't want to delve into the ins and outs of mastectomies, insurance copayments, and what her diagnosis would mean to their children, whom she didn't want to burden with all the details.

Knowing how intricately intertwined mind and body are, I recognized that she was compromising her already weak immune system by keeping a lid on her emotions. Healing an illness like cancer takes not only takes radiation and chemotherapy, but also an open mind to process the diagnosis and all the uncomfortable uncertainty that goes with it. You certainly don't have to embrace a potentially terminal illness, but you do have to acknowledge that you're in a murky, terrible place and, given that, allow yourself to grieve; otherwise, as I discussed in chapter 3, your unspoken anxiety can be as debilitating as the disease itself. "Unexpressed emotions tend to stay in the body like small ticking time bombs," writes Dr. Christiane Northrup in *Women's Bodies, Women's Wisdom*.[2]

Prompted by a lack of appetite and piercing migraines before she even started treatment, Teri mustered the courage during a consultation with an oncology nurse to mention how frightened she was. The nurse's first suggestion? Start a journal, since she had seen the writing process ease the emotional hearts of many patients before Teri. "Buy one with a beautiful cover and use the type of pen you like to write with," instructed the nurse. She then explained that expressing—and seeing—the feelings that Teri had swirling inside of her would help her come to terms with them, and, in doing so, set her emotional heart on the course she needed to heal her whole body.

Teri, sobbing for the first time since her initial diagnosis, drove immediately from the hospital to a stationery store and treated herself to a journal with an abstract bird design on the cover ("I paid $25 for essentially a notebook, but it was worth it," she admits) and an accompanying $20 fountain pen, along with ink refills. She went home and immediately sat down at her kitchen table. Her first entry, which started with the simple words "I have cancer," went on for seven full pages. She wrote (and continued to cry) for over an hour. "I could write what I couldn't say out loud," she remembers. "I put all my biggest fears out there. That I would die. That my husband would leave me. That I'd suffer for years and years. That I wouldn't be able to live a normal life."

By articulating her worst-case scenarios, she was able to face them directly and realize for the first time that she could handle them. The relief was like the quiet aftermath of a severe thunderstorm you've heard about over and over on the news. Finally, the sky grows darker and darker, the storm arrives, lights up the sky and shakes your world, and then passes and all is calm. The journal brought that serenity to Teri's heart. Although she knew she had plenty to weather as she healed her cancer, seeing on paper what storms were looming inside her made them less intimidating and quieted her mind. She wrote in her journal almost daily during her bout with cancer, and, in doing so, was able to spend her energy understanding her treatments, not fretting about the unknown.

Now cancer-free, Teri is the first person to recommend that anybody use pen and paper when faced with an unsupportive spouse, a lost job, a miscarriage, or any other life challenge. "I honestly believe my journal was a huge part of my healing," she says.

How we communicate with ourselves and others—or choose not to—is often underestimated when it comes to its effect on physical health. And I'm not just talking a failure to voice emotions when faced with challenging events. I'm referring to ways in which we communicate, in this digital world, nearly every second. How you voice your concerns on a group project with your coworkers. How you say (or don't say) good morning to your husband. How you respond to an abrasive email from your sister. How you approach a touchy topic with your adult children. How you praise or reprimand yourself. How you text on your BlackBerry when you're at dinner with a friend.

All those scenarios, depending on how they play out, can significantly influence your health. Do you avoid responding to your sister's email and bristle all day as a result? Chances are, you may overeat later in the day to diffuse your anger. Do you become confrontational with your adult kids when they bring up a potential caregiver? Your words may break down a dam, letting stress hormones flood your body. Do you read every email on your iPhone as it comes in, ignoring the world around you? Your blood pressure may pay the price for your fixation on digital messages.

Certain social rules widely govern how we communicate—look people in the eye when you talk to them, for instance—but nuanced, specific guidelines that take etiquette, emotions, and physical health into consideration are hard to find. Still, some scientific evidence indicates that the link between the messages you send to yourself, others, and the world at large has an effect on your health.

Communicating with Yourself

The internal conversation we have with ourselves is the most important communication we have on a daily basis because the way you talk to yourself is, most likely, the way you speak to others and the subliminal messages you send to the world.

On any given day, how many of your thoughts are positive? Negative? Putting a number to them might prove difficult, but, in general, do you dwell on failure, the things that you regret, relive the situations that put you on defense? Or do you do your best to move past the speed bumps we all encounter and celebrate the small victories, like no line at Starbucks or a good conversation with a tricky boss? Sounds trite, but the implications are massive. As Dr. Deepak Chopra is often quoted as saying, wherever a thought goes, a chemical goes with it. In other words, you may believe a negative thought like "I really hate my sister-in-law" is just an idea in your mind, when in reality, it jolts through your body. The idea of spending time with her may release cortisol, the stress hormone, and start your heart beating faster and your blood pressure soaring.

The brain's response to emotions has been studied in depth, and several studies indicate that how you process your life and yourself tends to promote thoughts, actions, and feelings in a similar vein. For seven years, researchers at the University of Texas at Galveston studied the link between positive emotions and frailty in almost 1,600 seniors. The participants who repeatedly answered yes to statements like "I enjoy life" and "I am hopeful about the future" lost less weight (a good thing, in your later years), had better grip strength, and maintained faster walking speeds than those who didn't have such a sunny outlook.[3]

Similarly, a study out of the Universities of Minnesota and Kentucky followed 180 nuns for six decades. Upon entering the convent, each nun was asked to write an autobiographical sketch describing how they internally processed the events of their lives. Despite leading remarkably similar lives and practicing similar health habits— they ate basically the same meals, for instance, and had similar daily schedules—the nuns who illustrated their life stories with positive statements and optimism were far more likely to live longer than those who had a negative outlook. A full 90 percent of the happiest nuns were still alive at age eighty-five, compared to a mere 34 percent of the least sanguine.[4]

The journal that helped Teri heal is also a scientifically sound strategy. A study out of the University of Kansas followed sixty women with early-stage breast cancer who were divided into three groups: one group wrote their deepest thoughts and feelings about cancer; one wrote only about the positive aspects of their experience; and the final group only wrote the facts about their treatment. After three months, the group who wrote about their full range of emotions reported markedly fewer negative physical symptoms than the other groups and had significantly fewer doctor visits for cancer-related issues.[5]

Rx for Better Doctor-Patient Communication

When it comes to your health, the most important conversations you will have will be with your doctor; it's vital that you have an open, honest, comfortable relationship with him or her. The more open the lines of communication are between you and your health care providers, the more likely you'll be motivated to take care of yourself. A study at Texas State University in San Marcos analyzed 127 studies that involved physician communication and patient adherence to treatment and found that patients of doctors who communicate poorly are 19 percent less likely to follow their instructions compared to those whose doctors communicate well.[6]

Communication goes both ways, of course. Observing my patients' experiences over time, I've developed a list of tips that can help you improve communication both during and following our office visit:

1. Bring a clear list of the symptoms that brought you to the doctor. If possible, write down pertinent details, like that the symptom happens "only at night," "after I eat dinner," "before I take medication," or similar notes. Often people forget the details when they're in my office.

2. Bring a list of specific questions you'd like answered and don't be afraid to ask questions, especially with regard to medication.

3. Bring a list of your current medications, including any supplements or herbal preparations you are using, even if you're only using them occasionally.

4. Also bring a list of any medical allergies and the side effects that led to the discontinuation of the medication.

5. Keep records of all your important tests, if you can. If you don't have the results and they aren't immediately available to your health care provider through an electronic record, make arrangements to have your prior evaluations and tests forwarded to the doctor you're currently seeing.

6. If possible, bring a family member or friend to take notes and record the discussion. It's very easy to get distracted during a visit, particularly with a new provider, and forget important items. I can't overemphasize how important this is: the most helpful and productive visits I have are when there's a third person in the room.

7. Ask if the doctor has access to a patient communication tool through the electronic medical record. It's a great way to order prescriptions, send messages to your practitioner, and give them feedback regarding your progress on a new medication, diet, or exercise program.

8. If you leave the appointment wanting more information or not liking the style of the doctor you saw, don't be afraid to find a new one. "You are the consumer. If you bought a coat and something was wrong with it, you'd bring it back," says health coach Cathy Culhane-Hermann. "If the doctor isn't giving you the time or answers you want, she or he isn't the right one for you. You are paying for [these] services. You have to be respectful, of course, but remember that you are in charge."

Communicating with Others

We've all had a conversation with somebody who has a virtual force field around herself. No matter what you say, you can tell she has a predetermined opinion and response, and she usually starts spitting it out before you even have a chance to finish your sentence. It's not a fun situation to be in—in fact, you usually walk away frustrated and probably with a not-too-favorable impression of the person.

We've also all had a conversation with somebody with whom you feel instantly connected. She "gets" you, a fact she transmits through her words, the way she talks with her eyes, her "uh-huhs," and other small comments at appropriate points. Those are the conversations you want to last forever because you walk away feeling energized and validated.

What's the difference between the two scenarios? Listening and then responding. Truly listening is a skill I'm still trying to perfect. My brain, just like yours, is wired to make snap judgments. Case in point: Dutch scientists asked people to listen to sentences coming from unexpected speakers—for example, "If only I looked like Britney Spears," spoken in a male voice or "I have a large tattoo on my back," said with an upper-class accent—and the brain responded to the speaker's identity in as little as 200 milliseconds. "Listeners rapidly classify speakers on the basis of their voices and bring the associated social stereotypes to bear on what is being said," explained the researchers.[7] Faster than you can blink your eye, your mind makes judgments about a speaker based solely on his or her voice and your perspective.

While I never discount friendly chatter, the depth of the conversation also matters. If you're going to ask an acquaintance "What's going on?" be willing to truly listen to the response and follow up with appropriate questions. (Obviously, this has its limits: "How are you?" can also be a nice, quick greeting to a stranger or a friend quickly passing.) Still, if you've got time for an engaging, interesting conversation, your health will benefit. According to early research by Matthias Mehl, a psychologist at the University of Arizona, the more substantive your conversations, the happier you'll be. Research on nearly eighty people who wore a voice recorder for four days showed that almost half of the conversations the happiest person had were meaningful, while only 21 percent of the unhappiest person's conversations were substantive.[8] Mehl is now researching whether people can actually make themselves happier by having more substantive conversations.[9]

Since we're talking about substance, I want to mention the ways of communicating with a keyboard: email, Facebook, blogging, texting, instant messaging, Twitter, and the like. What the digital world gains in efficiency, it can lack in personal connection. Typing on a keyboard is not the same as a face-to-face conversation. While the Internet has been great for connecting people and finding others with issues and conditions similar to yours, it's no substitute for being out in the world among people. Our HAPPY Heart women know this intimately; so many of them lived isolated, screen-centric lives until we brought them together. Now they're extremely close—all of them mention laughing together as the best part of the group—and have forged friendships they'll have for the rest of their lives. I'm positive it's because they got together and were able to see, touch, hug, and laugh with one another. Real laughter is much more meaningful than a smiley face on an email.

Research on the implications of email communication back up this idea. One study out of New York University found that conveying emotion is naturally difficult over email since vocal and physical cues like gesture, emphasis, and intonation are absent. "People tend to believe they can communicate over email more effectively than they actually can," write the authors.[10] In addition, another study found that people engaged in email communication, compared to those in face-to-face communication, were less likely to be cooperative and felt more justified in being noncooperative.[11]

Do-It-Yourself Internet Diagnosis

In a study released in 2010, researchers at Carnegie Mellon University in Pittsburgh looked at the effect of turning to the Internet for health-related reasons compared to more social reasons. It's one thing to use the Internet to figure out how to take care of a simple condition like head lice or a hangnail; it's another to self-diagnose a handful of symptoms, like headaches, fatigue, or muscle aches, that could be interpreted in a variety of ways, from the benign to the very serious.

Using a panel survey of 740 individuals who answered questions about their Internet use, health history, and depression levels, the team concluded that using the Internet for health-related reasons was associated with a, "small, but reliable increase in depression," while using it to stay in touch with family and friends had the opposite effect. "The increase [in depression] may be due to increased rumination, unnecessary alarm, or over-attention to health problems," write the authors in the conclusion.[12]

I can personally attest to this data. While living in Nova Scotia prior to starting my work at the hospital, I was fairly stressed. My husband was busy working in his fellowship, the children were all under four, and I was in a new location without the support of local friends and family. I developed tension headaches and started looking on the Internet. Even as a board-certified internist and cardiologist, I had convinced myself within hours of my Internet foray that I was suffering from multiple sclerosis.

When you have fears and anxiety about a medical illness, you can find information on the Internet that validates your fears. I have nothing against my patients being as fully informed as possible about their health, but I want them to get their information from safe, reputable websites. Here are some tips to make sure your information searches lead you down the correct path:

- **Be certain you are specific about the question you are asking and don't jump to any conclusions.** A patient of mine called me in tears after she looked up mild swelling in her feet. Based on the information she found, she thought the blood vessels to her feet were entirely blocked and she would need surgery. Turns out, the swelling was a benign, albeit annoying, side effect of a new medication.

- **Look for a sponsor or advertising.** If either are there, chances are, the information might have a bias toward the person funding the site.

- **If the address ends in .gov, .org, or .edu, it's a government agency, a professional organization, or an educational organization, respectively.** The information from such places is typically reliable. Addresses that end in .com or .net can be from anybody or any company; the information presented on those sites may be biased and may actually be a form of advertising. (For instance, www.diabetes.org is the American Diabetes Association; www.diabetes.com is funded by GlaxoSmithKline, a pharmaceutical company.)

- **Look for a revision or published date.** Health information is constantly changing, so you want the information to be current and relevant.

- **The information presented should be easy to read and be documented.** You should be able to tell, either by clicking on it or by a list of footnotes at the end, where the information came from.

- **A website that requires either your personal information or payment from you so you can use it is not reputable.** Do not give either.

Communicating with the World

There's a way you send messages to the world that doesn't involve your vocal cords. Your body language, which includes posture, hand gestures, facial expressions, and your perception of personal space speaks volumes to everybody from strangers to your loved ones.

Before delving too far into how you nonverbally interact with the world, I want to reemphasize that you need to do your best to be a part of the world. As I talked about in the loneliness section of chapter 7, isolation has powerfully negative effects on your health. An innovative project at the University of Chicago is currently studying 220 African-American women in an effort to uncover their predisposition to early-onset breast cancer compared to other populations. One reason, they speculate, is that they live, by and large, in poor neighborhoods where crime is prevalent. "They're stressed and afraid to go out, and are not able to form casual relationships with their neighbors that might make them feel safe," explained Sarah Gehlert, PhD, the lead researcher.[13]

A smile, it turns out, can be a big predictor of your fate. Scientists at DePauw University studied photos of people when they were around age ten and a separate group of people in their college yearbooks. In both cases, those who smiled most vigorously—toothy, genuine grins—had the happiest, longest-lasting marriages. "Those who smiled least were five times more likely to get divorced," lead researcher Matt Hertenstein, PhD, explained, stating that the more in touch you are with your emotions, the more you're able to share your life.[14] A similar study, out of Wayne State University in Michigan, tracked 230 major league baseball players, looking at their faces on their official pictures from the 1952 Baseball Register. Using death certificates, they concluded that those who weren't smiling died at the average age of 72.9, while those who had the biggest smiles lived an average of 79.9 years old.[15]

When it comes to nonverbal communication—or how your posture, eye contact, and facial expressions, among other things, also send a message—pioneering research by Albert Mehrabian, PhD, now Professor Emeritus of Psychology at UCLA, suggests that nonverbal communication is the gold standard. When you're talking about something that involves a feeling or attitude, only 7 percent of the message is conveyed in the actual words that are spoken; 38 percent is conveyed in the way in which the words are said; and a whopping 55 percent is conveyed in the facial expression.[16]

· The other point I want to address in this section is that simply the way you look may interfere with how others perceive you. Unfortunately, bias and prejudice still run rampant in our society, so somebody may judge you on the color of your skin, the size of your waist, the car that you drive, that you are a woman, and so on. Be aware of the biases, which are often unconscious, that exist in your life and address them accordingly.

The medical field is no different than the rest of the world. As a powerful woman in the male-dominated medical field, I encounter some form of judgment on a daily basis. Fine examples are the letters of recommendation written for female medical trainees. Women are frequently described using terms like *caring, warm, supportive,* while men are described with terms such as *intelligent, capable, talented.* The sad truth is that women supervisors are just as likely as their male counterparts to use this descriptive language. It's not fair but it's reality.

It's vitally important that you respect yourself enough to take care of yourself despite how others may think of or react to you. Researchers out of Drexel University College of Nursing and Health Professionals looked at the effect of the obesity stigma (defined as "a mark or token of infamy, disgrace, or reproach") on caring for people with type 2 diabetes. Looking at fourteen years of literature, they found that the stigma can often act as a barrier to management of the diabetes; some patients internalize the stigma so deeply, they avoid going to the doctor and getting the care they need.[17] If you have weight issues or other things that might elicit a preconception, stand up for yourself. If a doctor's staff treats you in an unprofessional or judgmental way, mention it to the doctor; if the doctor herself does, find a new practitioner. Don't sacrifice your health for somebody else's prejudice. (That said, a doctor is obviously there to help you improve your health. There are sensitive, helpful ways to encourage you to lose weight, stop smoking, or otherwise improve your health. "We don't let up on important messages, just because you might not be ready to hear them," says my colleague Kate Traynor, "but there are positive ways to impart the messages.")

Building the Bridge to Better Communication

Communicating with a happy, strong heart doesn't require a class in public speaking or a dramatic change in how you present yourself. Small shifts in your perspective can make huge changes in the way you respond to people and how they, in turn, react to you. Here are a few things I always keep in mind.

Turn Off the No's

If your self-talk is full of accusations ("You're so stupid: of course that happened") or criticisms, you need to start with shutting off that unhelpful chatter. Chances are, your body has somehow internalized that perspective, and you may pay for it with everything from insomnia to heart disease. What's more, thought loops are self-fulfilling—if you think you're going to lose, you probably will—and repetitive; negative thoughts beget unhappiness and poor health choices, while positive ones bring a sense of contentment and calm. When you find yourself headed down the negativity highway, it is a good idea to turn the car around and focus on something that brings you joy, fulfillment, or happiness. Let the negativity evaporate and then readdress the issue with a determination that you won't allow it to bring you down.

Listen First

As I mentioned before, listening is the key to great communication. My first goal is to go into any conversation, whether it's with a patient, a friend, or one of my children, with an empathic and positive approach. I want them to know that I'm focused only on them and that I am hearing and processing their words. I eliminate as much distraction as I can: no clicking a pen in my pocket, no checking my BlackBerry. I'm facing them and looking them in the eye. I ask plenty of questions and often repeat a short summary of what they said to me before I add ideas of my own, so that their feelings are validated and they know they've been heard.

Don't Interrupt

Habitual interruption of conversation gives the strong message to others that you are not listening to them and that what they have to say is not really important. This habit can undermine even the most jovial and lighthearted conversation and lead to anger and resentment, both of which have ties to an increased risk of heart disease.

Collaborate

My son with Asperger's syndrome has enhanced my communication skills. While most parents take it for granted that their child will look them in the eye or acknowledge their presence when spoken to, my son had to be taught and constantly reminded to look others in the eye when they are speaking to him and to listen when spoken to. We participated in a year-long program dedicated to helping improve his socialization and behavior. One of the tools we used is *collaborative problem solving*, which was developed by Dr. Ross Greene. When particularly difficult conversations come up with my son or anybody from another doctor to a friend, I use Dr. Greene's basic three-step approach:

1. **Be empathetic and reassuring.** Simply letting the other person know that you see where she is coming from is invaluable, and it often leads to a solution without much confrontation. In addition, ask appropriate questions, both objective and subjective, like What happened or is happening? Why do you feel this way? Why is this time different than the last time? Reassure the other person that you're not going to just dictate what happens in this situation.

2. **Lay out your own expectations and perspective.** In a calm voice, explain where you are coming from and how you see this problem.

3. **Come to a common solution that involves both of your input.** The resolution should be agreeable to both of you.[18]

Document

Like Teri discovered, a journal is one of the best ways to monitor both your internal and external conversations. You can run through your day in your head on your commute home or while you exercise, but putting pen to paper is invaluable. The visible record of your emotions, issues, and celebrations will not only give you something to reference if you find yourself in a similar situation in the future, but will also help you celebrate your achievements, cross off tasks, and prioritize your challenges. If a journey feels like too much of a commitment, just jotting down goals on a daily organizer is an easy place to start.

Stay Calm and Collected

When a difficult conversation comes up or the person with whom you're speaking is losing his or her cool, the first thing you should do is take a few deep breaths. Calm down your physiological system so that you're able to minimize the fight-or-flight syndrome. If you need to, excuse yourself from the conversation with a simple statement like, "I need some time to think about this" or "I'll be happy to continue this conversation at a later time when emotions aren't running so high." Very little good ever comes out of verbal conflict, so do your best to deflect it before it can begin.

Cut Yourself Off

Constantly responding to emails enforces reactive rather than proactive behavior; you aren't in control. If your iPhone is permanently affixed to your hand, turn it off for at least twenty minutes daily when you'd normally have it on. In addition, check email at your desk only once an hour. Research conducted in 2005 at London's Institute of Psychiatry found that incessantly checking and instantly replying to email has serious consequences; workers who were constantly on email alert suffered a ten-point fall in their IQ, which is more than twice what studies have found regarding the impact of smoking marijuana. What's more, the multitasking brains were as responsive as if they'd lost a night's sleep.[19]

Be Flexible

Recognize that no matter how hard you try or how much energy you expend, there will be others with whom you simply cannot communicate effectively. Some people build an invisible fence around themselves for protection and basically shut down. If you have tried to communicate more effectively, but nothing is happening, accept that you did your best and don't waste any more energy.

Three Easy First Steps Across the Communication Bridge

1. **Write a thank-you letter.** Not just a dashed-off note, it should be a thoughtful letter to somebody who has made a difference in your life: a friend, a teacher, a child, a relative. Give specific examples of why your life is richer and better because he or she left an imprint on it, and then send it. It's such a gift to find a handwritten note in the mailbox, and the effort required for you to write and then mail the note signifies the depth of your gratitude.

2. **Give one compliment daily.** It could be to your spouse, your kids, or a stranger. Forcing yourself to pay attention to small details about other people automatically draws you out of a self-centered, often downward-spiraling perspective.

3. **Smile.**

chapter nine

The Environment Bridge

One lifestyle examination that health coach Donna Slicis had the HAPPY Heart ladies do in a Monday night meeting was to dump out their purses. Like most women, the HAPPY Heart gang seems to carry around everything but the kitchen sink. On the tables, the voluminous piles contain everything from cough drops missing wrappers to pairs of socks to receipts from six months ago. "Look at what you carry around every single day," says Slicis—"How can you make room in your life for good things when you haul around all this unnecessary stuff?"

The metaphorical weight of hauling around unnecessary tubes of face lotion and receipts from months ago translates neatly to the often chaotic surroundings in the rest of their lives. What they—and you— surround yourself with is likely weighing on both your emotional and physical health. Case in point: Lisa, a HAPPY Heart participant, suffered from bad asthma. In the basement of her house was a pile of moldy towels. "She couldn't go down in the basement without suffering an asthma attack," remembers Slicis, "and yet she couldn't bear to throw the towels away." Her excuse was that she might need them one day to clean her car or house. Slicis turned the tables on her and asked her if it were her grandson that suffered from asthma, would she let him use the towels? "No way," Lisa replied. "Then why," asked Slicis, "would you let yourself use them?" Finally realizing a pile of old towels wasn't worth continually jeopardizing her health, Lisa washed them and donated them to an animal shelter.

We all have our own version of a moldy towel pile: some pile or issue in your surroundings that you know probably isn't good for you, but you continually either accept it—or at least fail to find the time or effort do to anything about. Maybe it's the stacks of papers you shuffle and reshuffle, but that never get any smaller—and the overdue bills that get lost in them. Could be the overstuffed pantry, which contains everything from wrenches to Oreos and is so crowded, you can't find any ingredients for a healthy dinner. Might be the pile of dusty books next to your bed.

While the study of environmental surroundings and health outcomes is exciting, it, like many other up-and-coming connections, is in its infancy. Still, it's pretty intuitive that your environment can affect your health. After all, we all can relate to how negative and unhealthy it feels to be in a dark room or cluttered space that is devoid of fresh air and natural light. I, for one, feel cramped, sad, and unmotivated. Those qualities—lack of light, stale air, piles of stuff—are things you can easily identify. And what about things you can't see or feel, like toxins? How might those be affecting your health?

Before you go any further, realize that I'm not going to go all Martha Stewart on you. I'm not asking you to totally redesign your house—or even make it spick-and-span. What I am asking you to do is consider how the places you spend the most time—your home, your car, your office—might be influencing your health, and then, if appropriate, start to make small changes that make these places more inviting and healthful. "It's amazing what you can do in fifteen minutes a day," says Lynne Johnson, a professional organizer and life coach in Quincy, Massachusetts. "If you just focus on those fifteen minutes, they add up to significant transformations at the end of a week, a month, a year."

So as I go through the five topics that I think are ripe for influencing your health—air quality, the natural environment, light, toxins, and clutter—remember that they, like everything else, are in your control, especially if you incorporate the easy changes I'll suggest at the end of this chapter.

Air Quality

Despite the recent appearance of this field, make no mistake: it is important. There's no doubt that the quality of the air we breathe plays into our overall health. A 2011 review published in *The Lancet* indicates the impact of air pollution: thirty-six previous studies about air pollution found it triggers nonfatal heart attacks at a rate similar to other previously established causes.[1] Other research shows that both short- and long-term exposure to air pollution, which is ubiquitous in most cities, contributes to causing and accelerating cardiovascular events.[2]

What might be surprising is that the air inside your house doesn't necessarily provide you with a safe haven from the pollution outside. The U.S. Environmental Protection Agency notes that "a growing body of scientific evidence has indicated that the air within homes and other buildings can be more seriously polluted than the outdoor air in even the largest and most industrialized cities."[3]

The quality of indoor air is far worse in developing countries where people heat homes with coal and wood; exposure to coal- and wood-based fires is very unhealthy. In 2006, I traveled to Tibet to work on a project that studied the effects of altitude on the hearts of Tibetan nomads. Working in a small room in a clinic that was heated by a coal stove, I could feel my lungs constricting and was sick within two days of arriving there.

The problems in the United States aren't as widespread, but they're definitely just as dangerous. Secondhand cigarette smoke is one the most toxic things you can breathe. Reams of research has shown that, when repeatedly exposed to secondhand smoke, nonsmokers are put at a higher risk of heart disease and stroke than people who aren't exposed to the fumes. In fact, breathing in the smoke of just one cigarette per day accelerates the progression of atherosclerosis in nonsmokers.[4]

Even though we know how dangerous secondhand smoke is, the research surrounding it continues to startle. Stating at the outset of a 2010 study that "there is no safe level of secondhand tobacco-smoke exposure," researchers at the University of Rochester investigated the effects of secondhand smoke exposure in children who lived with non-smokers in apartments, attached, and detached houses. Looking at levels of *cotinine*, a marker of secondhand smoke, they found that children who lived in apartments had cotinine levels that were 45 percent higher than those of their peers who lived in detached houses.[5] This study is particularly disturbing because while well-intentioned parents may refrain from smoking, their child can still be exposed to the detrimental effects of secondhand smoke.

Nitrogen dioxide, or NO_2, is another concern. The primary sources of NO_2 are cars, power plants, and other fossil-fuel burners. A handful of studies have pointed to a connection between NO_2 and cardiovascular disease. One, in 2005, found that inhaling high levels of diesel exhaust, typically found in large cities, has been found to disrupt normal blood vessel function and clotting, while another study, in 2007, suggested that long-term exposure to high volumes of traffic is associated with hardening of the arteries.[6] Indoors, the biggest sources of NO_2 are gas-burning appliances, like unvented furnaces and stoves, as well as kerosene space heaters and cigarette smoke. The American Heart Association notes that NO_2 levels may be higher indoors than outdoors, although it should be mentioned that a direct link between indoor NO_2 levels and cardiovascular disease hasn't been fully established yet.[7]

The Natural Environment

Nature is one of our most subtle, yet omnipotent healers; the positive effects of greenery have been well documented. In a comprehensive 2008 paper, Stephen Mitrione, MD, a family physician and landscape architect based in Minnesota, recounted the influence that natural environments can have on our health. "[Studies] show that all physiological measurements of stress (heart rate, blood pressure, muscle tension, and skin conduction) return to normal faster if the subject is allowed to recuperate in a natural setting as opposed to a man-made environment," Mitrione writes. "In addition . . . those same individuals had more positive feelings, experienced less fear, and showed less aggression in the natural environment." He then goes on to hypothesize that "natural environments interact with the central nervous system to reduce stress responses, which can favorably influence the outcome of diseases that are characterized by an overactivation of the stress response. This effect can be wide-ranging, producing changes in the endocrine, cardiovascular, and immune systems that have a positive effect on disease outcomes."[8]

I am a huge proponent of healing gardens. When I was going through radiation therapy for breast cancer, I would go to the garden at MGH and read EKGs. I found it much preferable to sitting in my sterile office. The environment, full of life and good smells, was very calming to me. Now, if I am going to have a difficult discussion with a family of a patient—perhaps we need to talk about withdrawing care—I prefer to have it in the garden on the cardiac rehabilitation floor. (We can close the door for privacy.) Although the scenery certainly doesn't soften the tough news, it definitely doesn't hurt to be in a vibrant, soothing place.

On a grand scheme, nature is one big calming bubble. Science has also begun to dive into the specifics about what particular aspects of the natural environment are most helpful. For example, in a 2009 study published in the *HortScience Journal*, four scientists screened twenty-eight plants for their ability to remove five common indoor *volatile organic compounds* (VOCs) commonly found in paint and household cleaners, among other things; VOCs have been linked to asthma and nausea as well as to chronic disease like cancer. They concluded that four plants—the *Hemigraphis alternata* (purple waffle plant), *Hedera helix* (English ivy), *Hoya carnosa* (variegated wax plant), and *Asparagus densiflorus* (Asparagus fern)—had the highest removal rates for all of the VOCs introduced.[9]

The Most Important Quality in Your Home

You can have the hippest furnishings in your living room and an amazing view from your kitchen, but if you don't feel relaxed in your own home, nothing will feel right. "Your home has to always feel safe," says Slicis, who adds that some of the HAPPY Heart participants say things like, "My house is safe except for when my husband drinks." That, obviously, is not acceptable. Living under constant threat of physical harm is certainly damaging to one's emotional and cardiovascular well-being. Your home should be your refuge. If it ceases to be, then you must make some tough but important changes. Domestic abuse or violence, which affects all classes and races, can range from humiliation and psychological abuse to financial abuse (withholding credit cards or money) to physical abuse. Any aspect of behavior that is threatening or abusive, whether it's a spouse, a child, or somebody else, in your home needs to be addressed for a variety of reasons, not the least of which is your health. Easier said than done, I realize, but please know that there are organizations that are equipped to handle domestic abuse or violence. A good place to start is the National Domestic Violence Hotline: 1-800-799-SAFE or www.thehotline.org.

Light

The value of being exposed to sunlight is priceless. Jennifer is one of the HAPPY Heart participants who suffers from *seasonal affective disorder*, a depression that coincides with the darker, cooler seasons of fall and winter. When the calendar turns to November, she seeks out the sun. "If the sun is out, I'm in it," she says with a laugh. "I used to drive down to the beach in the wintertime and park the car so the sun would shine in on me. I also sit in the bathhouse down at the beach— I know exactly where to sit so the sun can be on me—and read for a couple hours."

Although Jennifer's need for light is more intense than the average person's, people in the twenty-first century don't get as much time in the sun as we used to, and we're suffering because of it. Tall buildings block the sun's rays—and the amount of time we spend working inside them obviously doesn't do us any favors. Pollution, cars, and clothing also limit the amount of UVB rays that strike our skin.

The sun supplies our bodies with vitamin D, which is integral for healthy bones, muscles, nerves, and immunity. Low vitamin D levels have been shown to be associated with heart disease, cancer, and even sudden death. Your brain also benefits from sunlight. A 2009 study, out of the University of Alabama at Birmingham, looked at 16,800 participants, their cognitive function, and exposure to sunlight over a two-week period. The researchers found an association between decreased exposure to sunlight and decreased cognition.[10]

The Heschong-Mahone Group, an architectural consulting firm in California, has done extensive testing concerning light in different environments. They've tracked test scores of eight thousand third to sixth graders in Fresno, California; they've studied buying habits of consumers in chain stores lit by skylights; they've looked at cubicle culture and the effect that natural light—or lack thereof—has on work performance. Consistently, they concluded that the relationship between natural light and performance, which can be measured by worker satisfaction, test scores, or dollar amounts of sales, is an area that's ripe with possibility.[11]

A Place of One's Own

As I started to write this book, I realized that I did not have a space I could truly call my own in my home. While we have an office with a comfortable chair and desk, it is in high demand by my school-age children. So I retreated to my bedroom but found that writing while sitting at a cramped antique desk was actually detrimental to my productivity. I remember reading in Stephen King's book *On Writing* how important it is to have a comfortable, quiet environment in which to sow the seeds of creative thought.

Feeling like Goldilocks on the search for a place that was just right, I gave my dream workspace some thought. What I sought was an environment that evoked feelings of positive energy and creativity. The right mix of light, comfort, organization, and privacy to allow me the space to write. I found a lovely, warm, mission-style oak desk online for a song, got a very simple but elegant mission-style lamp (it was thrown in with the desk by the seller for a great price), a few plants and candles, and set about working. Now, whenever I need to, I can retreat into my own little world in the comfort of this space. I encourage you to create your own space too.

Toxins

One day, the media seizes on cell phones and the potential effects they have on your brain. The next day, baby bottles and the materials used to manufacture them make troubling headlines. There always seems to be another toxin hiding in some object, previously thought to be benign. And while it's important to pay attention to the controversies, the reality is, the research on what toxins get into our bodies and how they affect us is still spotty. Certainly, there have been materials that have been associated with—but not definitively linked to—an increased risk of cancer: pesticides, parabens (preservatives used in cosmetics and personal care products), and bisphenols (chemicals used to line cans and make plastics), among others, have all had their moments recently in the media spotlight. Although the deluge of news can be overwhelming, starting a gradual shift away from products that contain potentially toxic materials isn't as hard as you might think.

Move from conventional to organic produce, which can be affordably purchased throughout the summer months at farmers' markets; avoid or get rid of food containers that are not bisphenol free, especially for food storage and preparation; choose environmentally friendly toxin-free cleaning products.

Clutter

Most of the time, we have a picture of how we want our homes to be (clean, uncluttered, ready for a visitor at any moment), and then there's the reality (piles of mail, dust bunnies under the bed, yesterday's dishes still parked next to the sink). "You have to be realistic about what your life is like: if you have three small kids, two dogs, and work full-time, chances are, your house will look like you have three small kids, two dogs, and work full-time," says organizer Johnson.

So how do you know when you should address a mess? "If the mess keeps you from doing what you want to do, then it's time to think about making small changes," says Johnson. "If you're reading a book in the living room but can't relax because the piles of newspapers are bugging you, then it's time to clean. If you're always late in the morning because you can't figure out what to wear or where your keys are, then you need to get more organized. If you can't think straight because your office is full of clutter, then you need to sort through the piles."

More importantly, a lack of organization can get in the way of you leading a healthier life. "I have a lot of clients who are so frustrated because they lack the skills to plan out meals and grocery-shop productively," says Johnson, who notes that continually wanting to make changes but not having the infrastructure to do so will suck the energy and motivation out of you. When you know where your recipes are and what your pantry is lacking and have scheduled your day so you can take fifteen minutes to make a comprehensive grocery list, suddenly whipping up seven dinners this week doesn't feel akin to climbing a mountain.

And here's an unexpected health bonus to cleaning and clearing out your house: it'll help your stress levels (and not just because you'll know where you stashed your telephone bill). A study published in the *British Journal of Sports Medicine* that looked at nearly twenty thousand men and women showed that twenty minutes of housework a week (not a day) resulted in a significant reduction in stress and anxiety levels.[12]

Building the Bridge to a Better Environment

Unlike some of the other bridges that require some serious introspection and habit changes, there are plenty of simple, easy ways that you can clean up your environments. Here are some places to start.

1. To improve air quality

- **Test your house for radon gas.** If levels are above 4 picocuries per liter (pCi/L) or higher, you need to install a radon reduction system or consult a professional. For more information, check out www.epa.gov/radon/pubs/citguide.html.

- **Do not allow smoking in or near your house.** If possible, live in a detached house or a nonsmoking apartment complex.

- **Position carbon monoxide detectors near bedrooms.** Check them regularly to make sure they're functioning properly.

- **In rooms that have high humidity—bathrooms, kitchens, and basements—check for mold and make sure the rooms are properly ventilated.** The ventilation helps to prevent mold, which aggravates asthma and other pulmonary issues.

- **If you're concerned about your air quality, use an air purifier outfitted with high-efficiency particle air (HEPA) filter in the rooms you use the most, like your bedroom, kitchen, and living room.** When somebody lives in an environment that is not healthy—living with a smoker, in an apartment, in a house heated with wood or coal—research has shown that the machines do an effective job. A 2011 study out of British Columbia, where wood stoves are prevalent, found that using air purifiers with HEPA filters reduced the average concentration of fine particulates by 60 percent and wood smoke by 75 percent. In addition, looking at the cardiovascular health of forty-five individuals in twenty-five houses, the scientists found markers of improved efficiency in the cells that line the blood vessels and reduced inflammation.[13]

- **When you come in your house, leave your shoes at the door.** That way any pesticides or other outdoor contaminants are minimized.

2. To get more green

- **Try to have at least one plant in most rooms in your house.** If you have previously proven that you are lacking a green thumb, find low-maintenance plants, like cacti or hardy ivy.

- **Grow a garden.** If you live in an apartment or other situation where it isn't possible, look into community gardens or simply get a large pot for some tomatoes or flowers. Another option: Just grow your own herbs—a rewarding and healthy endeavor. Snip your own chives, basil, or thyme and use them to flavor your cooking. Spend more time outside. Sounds simple, but it can be hard to do with a busy day. Take your lunch break outside; instead of going to the gym, head to a park and exercise there; ride your bike to the grocery store instead of driving.

- **Challenge yourself to learn more about a plant you like but have never had the courage to attempt to grow.** Read online about orchids, African violets, or flowering plants and get to work. The simple act of learning something new, putting that knowledge into action, and getting to enjoy the end results will do wonders for you.

3. To maximize natural light

- **If you've got heavy curtains on your windows, consider switching to loosely woven light colors or blinds.** You'll still have privacy, just not as much darkness.

- **Move furniture**—or anything else blocking a window— away from it.

- **Consider installing skylights.** A light that has a shape— arch, pyramid, or dome—captures and allows in more light than a flat-paneled one does.

- **Consider painting with a glossy, light-colored paint.** It creates the brightest atmosphere because gloss reflects more light than flat paint does.

- **Hang mirrors, especially on walls opposite big windows.** They'll throw natural light through the house.

- **Wash your windows.** It's a simple solution that makes a big difference.

- **Exercise outside when possible but always wear sunscreen.** The risk of skin cancer outweighs the benefit of vitamin D, in my mind. If you want to bare your skin to the sun, the National Institutes of Health notes that some vitamin D researchers have suggested that five to thirty minutes of sun exposure between 10 a.m. and 3 p.m. twice a week is sufficient for vitamin D synthesis. They also note, however, that, "people generally do not apply sufficient amounts [of sunscreen], cover all sun-exposed skin, or reapply sunscreen regularly. Therefore, skin likely synthesizes some vitamin D even when it is protected by sunscreen as typically applied."[14]

4. To minimize toxins

- **Try to keep foods, cleaning products, and food storage items as natural and basic as possible—and try to have as much control over what you eat, drink, and come into contact with as possible.** The lower you eat on the food chain, the fewer preservatives and chemicals you will come into contact with.

- **Use organic or toxin-free garden and cleaning products whenever possible.**

- **Buy organic foods.** I realize that this can be expensive. One way to mitigate the expense is to be choosy about what you buy organic and what you don't. The Environmental Working Group (ewg.org) has put together a list of the dirty dozen (the foods with the highest number of pesticides) versus the clean fifteen (the foods with the fewest).[15]

Dirty Dozen	Clean Fifteen
1. Apples	1. Onions
2. Celery	2. Sweet corn
3. Strawberries	3. Pineapple
4. Peaches	4. Avocado
5. Spinach	5. Asparagus
6. Nectarines (imported)	6. Sweet peas
7. Grapes (imported)	7. Mangoes
8. Sweet bell peppers	8. Eggplant
9. Potatoes	9. Cantalope (domestic)
10. Blueberries (domestic)	10. Kiwi
11. Lettuce	11. Cabbage
12. Kale/collard greens	12. Watermelon
	13. Sweet potatoes
	14. Grapefruit
	15. Mushrooms

- **Avoid cooking in plastic whenever possible.** If you're going to microwave foods, do it in glass or ceramic.

- **Filter your drinking water.** Bottled water, by the way, is not the way to go for myriad reasons, not the least of which is that it's not regulated.

- **Keep your grooming products as natural as possible.** In the ingredient list, if you see the words *paraben* or *phthalate*, two compounds that can disrupt hormones, don't buy it. The website cosmeticsdatabase.com, which is run by the Environmental Working Group, also has comprehensive information.

- **Keep your home as chemical free as possible.** Don't opt for extra stain treatment on your carpets or furniture; steer clear of air fresheners; use volatile organic compound (VOC)-free paint; ask if your dry cleaner uses perchloroethylene (perc), another VOC.

- **Finally, dust and vacuum weekly.**

5. To clear up clutter

- **Move things along.** Johnson isn't a huge fan of the touch-it-once philosophy, where you only handle an object once before putting it away totally. That perspective often invites doing nothing; if you're not going to get it to where it needs to be in one fell swoop, you are inclined not to handle it at all. Instead, suggests Johnson, move it along the path: get a bill into the right pile or move your dress shoes to the bottom of the stairs. "You might not be able to completely deal with it, but you can get it closer to where it needs to be."

- **Enroll an objective reviewer.** When you're cleaning out your closet, a basement full of memories, or anything else to which you're personally attached, ask a friend who isn't judgmental to help you distill what you need, what looks good on you, what you're holding onto simply because you feel you have to. "So many people buy things that don't work out but can't throw them away without feeling guilty," says Johnson. "Just because you acquired it doesn't mean you have to keep it." Donate to the library, the local women's shelter, Goodwill, or any other charity.

- **Create a landing and launching zone near the entrance of your home.** A small tray or basket can hold your keys, phone, sunglasses, and other essentials, while a larger mat and coat rack are great for your outer gear. "You can easily knock off a few minutes every morning by not running around looking for your things," says Johnson.

- **Take responsibility for the mess.** As Cindy Glovinsky, M.S.W., A.C.S.W., says in her book *One Thing at a Time*, "People often talk about things as if they're alive and trotting around on little legs . . . This kind of thinking . . . implies that you're a powerless victim upon whom your papers and possessions insist on ganging up."[16] Your clothes don't end up on the floor. You put them there. Papers don't pile up. You pile them up. As with all things in your life, asserting that you have control is key. Shift your thinking and take control.

- **But don't be a control freak.** If you live with your family, assign certain tasks to every family member, even young kids. "The younger you start to train them, the easier it is as they age," says Johnson. "I recently met with a mom who felt like she had to control everything. Unless her family owned part of the decision making, nothing was going to change."

Three Easy First Steps Across the Environment Bridge

1. **Simplify your life.** The less you have, the less you have to worry about. You don't have to live a spartan life, but if you have been described by friends or family as a "hoarder," recognize it is time for change. Bring on the purge patrol: a friend or family member who will help you part with your

stash. Starting with your kitchen, systematically go through and rid yourself of unnecessary bowls, jars, canisters, and canned or boxed items you have no intention of eating or using. Slowly move from room to room until you are surrounded by things you know you need.

2. **Clean with care.** A combination of vinegar and water is a great substitute for most mild household cleaners. When you need to use the heavier-duty stuff, like bleach, open a window and use gloves and a mask.

3. **Secretly regift.** Just because you were given something as a gift doesn't mean you have to keep it. If you don't like it or can't use it, discreetly pass it along to a friend who will use it or donate it to a shelter or Goodwill.

chapter ten

The Mindfulness Bridge

Susie has barely known a day in her life without pain because of a case of severe rheumatoid arthritis. She was diagnosed with the debilitating disease at age thirteen, but the official diagnosis was likely years overdue. "It wasn't really thought of as a disease for kids back then," says Susie, now fifty-three. Over the decades, the disease has ravaged her body and spirit; she regularly struggles with depression. "Constant pain really does a number on you," she says. Due to a lack of cartilage, she's had both knees and elbows replaced, as well as one hip. "I still need to get the other hip done," she says, "but the thought of another surgery is so overwhelming. I can't stand the recovery, not being able to drive and be independent."

Before she headed into another joint replacement surgery, Susie learned to do something so basic, yet so powerful, that her perspective changed nearly 180 degrees. Susie learned how to breathe deeply. "Turns out, I was breathing the wrong way my whole life," she says with a laugh. While she was obviously getting oxygen into her lungs, she wasn't enjoying the many benefits that deep, deliberate breaths bring to your body.

Susie learned how to alter her breathing in HAPPY Heart yoga classes, where she was introduced to the connection between the breath, mind, and body; when you breathe with intention, you quiet your mind and rejuvenate your body. Almost instantly, life doesn't feel so stressful and you don't feel so out of control—sounds too good to be true, I realize, but just ask Susie: it's not. Out of class, she took time on her own to focus on her breath, consciously slowing down the inhales and exhales as much as possible. Sensing how much calmer she felt immediately, she felt like she was getting a new life skill with no instructions necessary. "I take deep breaths all the time now," she says—"when I'm driving, when I'm at the grocery store, when I'm going to sleep. I deal with stress so much better now than I've ever been able to."

Susie didn't stop with yoga and her oxygen intake. She revamped many of her habits so that she could lower her stress and pain levels. She started listening to and following the instructions on relaxation CDs and drinking herbal tea before she went to bed. "A world of difference," she says. She also adopted a mantra, a simple phrase that she repeats when she starts to feel overwhelmed or needs to calm her focus. She simply repeats, "I am at peace. I am at peace. I am at peace."

Most of all, Susie has learned that she has much more control over her state of mind and her body than she ever thought possible—a great skill to have, especially because she prefers not to take pain medicine despite her multiple opportunities to use it. When she shifts her focus away from the pain and onto her breath and the accompanying sense of peace and relaxation, she is noticeably more comfortable. She's also learned how to easily bring joy into her life. "I've learned that just being outside relaxes me," she says. "I love planting flowers in the park or tomatoes at my house. They sound kind of silly, but I've learned that the little things make me feel so much better."

All the things that Susie thinks are little—breathing, a mantra, doing things that make you relax—are actually quite substantial and powerful. They, along with other methods that encourage reflection, a sense of tranquility, the ability to live in the present, and a sense of feeling grounded, make up the mindfulness bridge.

Sometimes our best moments occur when we are listening only to the sound of our breathing and feel that positive flow of energy that courses through our body when we are content, fulfilled, and totally mindful. What happened in the past seems inconsequential, and what the future holds isn't troubling; the present is, in a word, perfect. That inner nirvana can happen when holding a newborn child or grandchild, when practicing a difficult yoga pose, when kneeling in a church pew, or when flying a jet thirty-six thousand feet above the ground. I find this peace when I am reading to one of my children quietly at night, caring for my patients, or running alone with the wind in my face.

This introspective moment for each of us is unique and extremely personal; it's that place where we stop striving and struggling and instead simply exist and, in doing so, grow stronger. The mindfulness bridge is the place where we find our inner peace that allows us to tolerate all those moments in our life that do not necessarily come so easily or flow so nicely for us. I will go through the research as it relates to health and mindfulness and related practices, but remember that there is no one way to cross this bridge. Instead, there is simply a common goal at the end: a greater sense of self, connection, purpose, generosity, forgiveness, and serenity.

Meditation

The first thing that comes to mind with the word *mindful* is *meditation*, the practice of quieting one's mind through concentrated focus on one object, whether it be the breath, a saying, or an object. One of the most recent studies that examined the potential health benefits of meditation involved 201 African-American patients with coronary artery disease. Half of them practiced *transcendental meditation* (TM), a style of meditation that is described as a mental health relaxation technique, twice daily for twenty minutes a time for five years. The other half had simple health education programming. After the study was over, the group that meditated had cut their risk of heart attacks, strokes, and deaths from other causes by about half; over the course of five years, twenty in the meditation group had suffered a cardiac event while thirty-two in the comparison group did. What's more, the meditation group suffered less stress and reduced their systolic blood pressure by 5mmHg.[1]

The mental benefits of meditation are similarly remarkable. A group of researchers at MGH had sixteen participants take place in the mindfulness-based stress reduction class, an eight-week course that integrates *mindfulness meditation* (a type of meditation that centers on focusing) in a nonjudgmental way, on the present emotions and sensations your body is experiencing, and not fixating on thoughts about the past or future. They took MRIs of the participants pre- and post-course and compared those scans to people who didn't meditate. The scans, which documented for the first time physical changes due to meditation, showed greater density in the hippocampus, the part of the brain associated with learning and memory, as well as in parts of the brain that are connected to self-awareness, compassion, and introspection. The people who meditated also reported reductions in stress, which was correlated on the MRIs.[2] "By practicing meditation, we can play an active role in changing the brain and can increase our well-being and quality of life," said Britta Hölzel, PhD, the lead author.[3]

Meditation Resources

While there are plenty of books and articles that teach you how to meditate, I think it's important to have some verbal guidance, either in a class or via a video. An instructor will help you set the mood, focus your mind, and stay engaged. Here are some ways to get started:

- Look for beginner classes through your community center, local meditation center, or yoga studios.
- The HAPPY Heart group uses the Benson-Henry CDs for guided relaxation and meditation, which are available at www.mghgeneralstore.com.
- Many public libraries have DVDs or CDs you can borrow so you can sample different styles of meditation before settling on one.
- YouTube has a variety of resources, including a virtual mindfulness class led by Jon Kabat-Zinn, a professor emeritus of medicine at the University of Massachusetts and author of several books on mindfulness.

Prayers and Mantras

As Susie found out, mantras can indeed be very helpful in easing both the mind and body. Italian researchers had twenty-three healthy adults recite either the rosary prayer (Ave Maria in Latin) or a yogic mantra (om-mani-padme-om). They serendipitously found that both the prayer and the mantra caused, "striking, powerful, and synchronous increases" in cardiovascular rhythms, because both slowed the breathing rate to almost exactly six respirations per minute, which is essentially the same timing as a body's circulatory rhythms. In other words, the breath and the body were almost totally in sync; because of that, the researchers noticed enhanced heart rate variability and *baroreflex* (or blood pressure) sensitivity—two factors that can potentially contribute to heart disease.[4]

While the researchers concluded that sayings that prompt you to breathe six times a minute induce positive psychological and possibly physiological effects, there's no need to break out a timer and get technical about it. Any saying or prayer that calms your mind and slows your breath is beneficial.

Music and Art

In 2009, researchers at Temple University in Philadelphia analyzed the results of twenty-three previous studies that looked at the effect that music had on patients with coronary heart disease (CHD). Although they noted that more research needs to be done, they concluded that "music listening may have a beneficial effect on blood pressure, heart rate, respiratory rate, anxiety, and pain in persons with CHD."[5]

One year later, Dr. Hans-Joachim Trappe, a cardiologist and director of the Medical University Clinic at the University of Bochum in Germany and an accomplished church organist, compiled all the effects that music may have on the cardiovascular system and cardiovascular health. One study, he notes, showed that listening to music while resting in bed after open-heart surgery significantly reduces cortisol levels. "The greatest benefit on health is visible with classical music and meditation music, whereas heavy metal music or techno are not only ineffective but possibly dangerous and can lead to stress and/or life-threatening arrhythmias," he writes. "The music of many composers most effectively improves quality of life, will increase health and probably prolong life, particularly music by Bach, Mozart, or Italian composers."[6]

While Trappe's findings about classical music are interesting, Italian researchers came to a different conclusion about music. They designed a study to gauge the effect of a variety of styles of music, as well as silence, on blood pressure, heart rate, and breathing rate, among other things, in twenty-four people: twelve trained musicians and twelve regular people. They used music from Beethoven, Vivaldi, Red Hot Chili Peppers, sitar music, techno music, and dodecaphonic orchestral music. The biggest finding they found was that the tempo of the music was the one thing that dictated cardiovascular effects. Fast music made listeners' blood pressure, heart, and breathing rates go up, while slower music brought those things down accordingly.

The biggest finding, though, was that silence was the most effective at calming the cardiovascular system. A two-minute silence in the middle of the music brought down heart rate and blood pressure more significantly than slow music.[7] "The silence had a totally different effect on heart rate and other parameters when it came after music than it did at baseline," Dr. Bernardi told the journal *Circulation*. "Silence between music had the most profound relaxing effect." He compared it to meditation. "First, you have to concentrate hard, giving your attention to something. Then, when you release the attention, you become very relaxed," he said. "Music may be able to achieve the same effect."[8]

These studies, taken together, suggest that the genre of music that leads to this relaxation may differ from person to person. Listen to several types of music—try everything from an opera to new age music—to find the type of music that allows you to drift and totally relax.

Art therapy, like drawing and painting, seems also to bring on beneficial effects. Analyzing studies that looked at the connection between patients with cancer and art therapy, German researchers saw trends that included an increased quality of life, less anxiety and depression, better coping skills, and enhanced personal growth.[9] While that study focused on cancer patients, anybody can benefit from creative expression and stimulation of part of the brain you may normally not use. Plus, a bonus is you end up with a piece of art that is reflective of your efforts.

Yoga

Yoga, a centuries-old practice that unites breath with movement, is profoundly helpful when it comes to being mindful and healthy. One study out of the Mayo Clinic in Rochester, Minnesota, put fifty coworkers on an intense, brief yoga program: they practiced yoga for an hour a day, six days a week for six weeks. (Just so you know, life still gets in the way of studies: only thirty-seven of them made it to more than 90 percent of the classes.) In addition to the yoga postures, the classes also integrated other mind-body exercises like journal writing and mindful eating. At the end of the six weeks, there were improvements in all the physical markers (weight loss, lower blood pressure and body fat, better flexibility) as well as quality of life.[10]

Yoga is as beneficial for people whose health isn't ideal. Living with chronic disease associated with pain, like fibromyalgia, can be very difficult, as this type of illness can affect every aspect of one's life. (I see many women who suffer from fibromyalgia because it often overlaps with other symptoms, including chest pain.) Researchers in Oregon put half of a group of fifty-three females who suffered from fibromyalgia on an eight-week Yoga of Awareness program, which included gentle poses, meditation, breathing exercises, yoga-based coping instructions, and group discussions, and the other half on standard care. The group who took yoga showed bigger improvements in pain and fatigue levels, and mood, as well pain acceptance and coping strategies.[11]

Similarly, Australian researchers put stroke victims on a ten-week yoga program and found that, postprogram, the participants felt stronger and calmer and were more open to reconnecting and accepting their new, different bodies.[12] The latter benefit—realizing and being kind toward a body that isn't as healthy as you'd like it to be—is especially notable, as many women with cardiovascular disease could be mentally in the same space. As I talked about in the emotional health bridge, there's a barrier between health and unhealth, and when you cross it due to heart disease or other significant diagnosis, yoga can be a great tool for mentally reconciling your situation.

How to Breathe Deeply

The beauty of using your breath to control your mood and stress levels is three-fold: First, it's always available. Second, it's free. Third, you are already familiar with the motion.

You do have to put a little thought into it, but it's one of the simplest exercises in this book. Here's a five-step process to finding your calming, relaxing breath:

1. First, just tune into your breath: notice the sensations of your body as you inhale and exhale.

2. After a few breaths, focus on the inhale. Breathing through your nose, aim to fill up your abdomen with air; the oxygen should feel like it's inflating all of your lungs, not just the top portion.

3. As you exhale through your nose, send the air out of your belly by pulling your navel toward your spine.

4. As you breathe with intention, slowly lengthen each inhale and exhale so that they are roughly the same length.

5. Do your best to keep your mind focused on your breath. If your focus strays, don't fret: just take a deep breath and get back on track.

Tai Chi

When I first visited China in 2000, I noticed how robust the elderly practitioners of tai chi, a martial art that uses gentle movements that create a meditative state, were. They piqued my interest because I strongly believed in the untapped healing potential of the mind-body connection—and I wanted to try to validate one aspect of it. I set out to determine whether tai chi, which has been practiced for thousands of years, could provide any benefits for patients with heart failure. (I picked heart failure because it is one of the most common diseases I encounter, and for good reason: five million men and women suffer from heart failure in the States and it is the number one cause of disability in women.)

To show that tai chi was safe—and potentially helpful—for sick patients with congestive heart failure, we started with a pilot program. We recruited thirty patients with chronic systolic heart failure and enrolled them in a twelve-week tai chi program: they'd do tai chi together twice a week, plus practice on their own at home using tapes. Compared to a control group that didn't do tai chi, the ones who practiced the martial art saw great improvements in quality of life, exercise *self-efficacy* (the ability to initiate participation in exercise), and overall mood.[13] The quality-of-life aspect stood out for me most; patients with heart failure are unable to do many activities they enjoy, including exercise, because of symptoms like profound fatigue and shortness of breath.

Tai chi helped the patients because it ratcheted down their bodies' fight-or-flight response, which is revved up in heart failure. The ability to open up the healing energy trapped within them and direct it to areas of need within their bodies likely also contributed to the benefit. These findings were subsequently verified in a larger study, which included one hundred patients.[14]

Building the Bridge to Mindfulness

One of the easiest ways to be more mindful is to simply stop and ask yourself, "Am I paying attention to where I am now? To what I am doing at this very instant?" Chances are you aren't, especially if you're driving, emptying the dishwasher, or doing any other task you've done thousands of times before. A couple times a day, check in with yourself: are you present? Is your mind where your body is, or is it worrying about dinner tonight, an outstanding bill, or a sick friend? Caring about and addressing items like these is obviously important, but if they're constantly on your mind, they'll wear you down. Luckily, there are several ways to encourage yourself to be present.

Prioritize Yourself

If the message of taking care of yourself hasn't quite penetrated your psyche yet, here's another shot at it. You *must* take time for yourself to do things that bring you happiness and peace. From the start, one of the goals of the HAPPY Heart study was to provide women with structured "me time," in the form of our weekly meetings and exercise classes. We wanted them to realize the inherent value of this time so that they'd learn how to build more of it into their own lives. Thankfully, they have. They meet for coffee. They exercise. They read books. They take baths.

The hardest thing about me time is that it doesn't just organically appear. You've got to consciously carve the time out of your schedule; start with thirty minutes daily, and as you begin to adjust and appreciate that, bump it up to an hour in small increments. Once you've got your time figured out, stick to it: don't let a lack of motivation or another commitment eat into it. I find that early morning or later in the evenings works best for me: in the mornings, nobody else is awake, and in the evenings, I enforce an 8:30 bedtime for kids with no exceptions.

Find a Hobby

One easy way to enforce me time is to cultivate a hobby: could be knitting, painting, learning an instrument or a new language. Creative expression is a great way to decompress and relax. I enjoy reading, playing the piano, and running. I find playing a musical instrument both refreshing and challenging. It forces me to use parts of my brain that otherwise are "hibernating" and always leaves me feeling intellectually stimulated.

Get Your Om On

Yoga, which used to feel like it was only for the extremely limber and fit, is very much for the masses now. In fact, many of the HAPPY Heart women started with chair yoga, doing simple, small movements their bodies were able to do. They still reaped the benefits. "I wish everybody used yoga as a tool," says Susan. Beginner yoga classes are offered at community centers and gyms, and there are a variety of DVDs that can also guide you if you're feeling shy.

Expand Your Definition of Meditation

Certainly, the most accepted way to meditate is sitting down in a silent space. But that doesn't mean you have to do it that way. Lie down if you're most comfortable (although be aware that you may fall asleep). If you get too restless, try tai chi, which is often called meditation in motion. A walk or run on a quiet path can also be a meditative experience; you can repeat a mantra in rhythm to your footsteps. The goal of meditation is to give your conscious mind a break; training it to do so easily and regularly help you emerge from the practice energized and refreshed.

Try Tai Chi

My personal experience with tai chi backs up what we proved: it's powerful medicine. I attended and participated in the classes once a week, and over the course of time was able to recognize and appreciate the *qi*, or energy, that was stimulated during the practice. What's more, I clearly witnessed the benefits in the patients. One woman was very depressed, due to having to live with a disease with such a dire prognosis. She felt trapped in her home and body. Within weeks, I could see the life return to her eyes. She started driving again, getting out of her house and living.

Be Consistent

As with most healthy habits, practices like yoga and meditation are most fulfilling when you do them on a regular basis. Trying to meditate, in whatever form it may take, for one day, getting frustrated and then not trying again for another month isn't going to make a difference in your life. Instead, commit to most days of three consecutive weeks and just do it without judging the process. As little as ten minutes a day can set you on a path to better health. After you've been consistent for three or so weeks, look back and see if you're in a better place than you were when you started. Kara started with a twenty-minute mini-relaxation CD years ago, and now she's up to forty-five-minute sessions of meditation a couple times a week. "If I didn't meditate, I'd be in the loony bin," she says, half-joking. "It gives me a chance to zone out and recharge."

Three Easy First Steps Across the Mindfulness Bridge

1. **Slow down when you eat.** At your next meal, turn off any distractions—the phone, computer, TV, music—and simply eat. Put your fork down between each bite and do your best to savor the food in your mouth. Don't think about what you'll eat next or what you have to do tomorrow: simply enjoy the bite you have now.

2. **Get in the habit of taking deep breaths.** Pick a cue you see often, like a stop sign or stoplight, or every time you get an email at work. Before you push on the gas or click the mouse, take three, slow, diaphragmatic breaths through your nose.

3. **Ease up on the multitasking.** When you're doing a task, do your best to focus simply on that task and not on others or what's coming up. Instead of emptying the dishwasher as you talk on the phone, sit down and digest the conversation. Instead of watching television and checking email, do one or the other.

chapter eleven

The Modification Bridge

When asked what her goals are for the upcoming year, Heather, the HAPPY Heart participant who got new knees, a dog and, with them, a new life, doesn't hesitate. "I want it to be about me," she says, not at all self-conscious about how others might perceive that statement as egotistical. "I don't mean to be selfish, but my life has never been about me. It's always been about my family and their needs. It's finally my turn to take care of myself."

Taking Care of Yourself

Now it's your turn to take care of yourself—and your health. With nine bridges already addressed, your own HAPPY Heart toolbox is overflowing with information, ideas, and possibilities. Modification, the tenth and last bridge, is the hardest one, as it requires you to put your tools to work so you can become truly smart at heart.

But before we go into the fine details of how to change your habits for the better, I want you first to close this book, take a moment and some deep breaths, and, as you center your mind, give yourself a pat on the back for two things. First of all, congratulate yourself for picking up this book. That simple choice suggests that you are looking and ready to make some changes to enhance your physical and emotional well-being. Don't underestimate how important that step was.

The second bit of recognition comes for making it to chapter 11. Presumably, you've gone through the previous nine bridges, and even though some of the specifics may have felt daunting, you've stuck with it and now you're here. Now, just a little more guidance and a continued optimistic attitude will set you on the smart-at-heart path.

Since I've already told you this is the hardest bridge, I may as well heap on a little more slightly challenging news: the smart-at-heart journey never ends. "You're always in action," says Kate Traynor, RN, MS, program director of the Cardiovascular Disease Prevention Center at the MGH. "There is no final step which brings you to ideal cardiovascular health. For the rest of your life, you'll be in maintenance mode."

While maintenance mode might sound onerous now, realize that each time you opt for a walk around the block instead of a cigarette, pick carrots instead of chips, or take a deep breath to defuse your anger instead of blowing up, you're setting yourself up for the choice to be easier and more natural next time. Eventually, it will get to a point where the daily decisions you make regarding your health will become so ingrained in your routine and subconscious that they'll feel almost effortless. Realigning your goals and your priorities will change the way you approach your day. If you want to exercise, to find time to spend on your new personal journey, you will need to be more efficient in the other activities that occupy your day. That efficiency will be likely to make you more productive and organized. It is amazing how once you get yourself moving and your blood pumping, your energy and enthusiasm levels respond accordingly.

So how do you get to the point where what can feel impossible today feels almost second nature in the future? Here are ten strategies that have worked for my HAPPY Heart participants and leaders, patients, and myself.

Realize That Your Someday Is Now

As far as I know, we all have one beautiful, precious life. If you wait for some exact right moment to start on the path to a healthier way of living, you'll likely be waiting for the rest of your life. Just as there's no perfect time to have a child or get married—all the complications of life in general continue, as your life becomes more complex—there's never a time where the seas part, and you are certain today is the day.

You may think that a heart attack or similar cardiac event might be enough of a motivator to solidify the call to action, but, unfortunately, it's not. "Many times people say, 'I'm so afraid, I'll never do that again,'" says Traynor, "but fear only lasts about a year as a motivator. The memory of the event fades and it alone won't be enough to keep you on track. Fear will get you started, but it won't sustain you." Your conscious choices are what sustain you.

Certainly there are easier times than others to concentrate on your own health, but the reality is this: if you don't take time today—not someday—not only are you likely shortening your life, you're also depriving yourself of a better quality of life.

Pick One Thing to Work On at a Time

"I've heard it so many times: 'I am going to do it all or I am going to do nothing,'" says health coach Donna Slicis. "That's the totally wrong perspective." What bridge feels most conquerable to you? That's the place to start. As you experience success, that positive feeling will be encouragement to progress to other bridges. Don't feel the need to tackle the bridges sequentially, in their chapter order—if a different order makes sense to you, go for it.

Then Take Small Steps

Despite what reality television shows or weight loss commercials may say, you're not going to lose fifty pounds in eight weeks. You're not going to be able to reconcile a tangled relationship with your parents in that time either. But what you can do is break down those ambitious goals into bite-size pieces. Switch out your glass of soda with dinner for water for one week, or add an apple to your snack so that you're not as inclined to eat junk food. Ask your mom for thirty minutes of uninterrupted conversation time each Saturday for a month. Those doable steps will give you the momentum you need to take additional steps; in due time, you'll have climbed the whole staircase.

And Celebrate Your Small Successes

There is no such thing as a feat too tiny to appreciate; every decision you make that is better than the one you would've made yesterday is a victory. In HAPPY Heart, we've celebrated participants eating one piece of cheesecake instead of the whole thing, dancing through six Zumba routines instead of having to take a break after one song, decreasing the number of cigarettes smoked daily from forty to thirty, and minimizing a draining friendship. "Sometimes when you're the one making the change, those small steps don't feel so positive," says Cathy Culhane-Hermann, one of the health coaches, "but in the scheme of things, it's a huge improvement."

Melanie's Story

Unlike the other patients cited in this book, Melanie is not a pseudonym. Melanie Harvey, also a patient of mine, is an ambassador for the Massachusetts chapter of the American Heart Association's Go Red for Women campaign. Here's her story.

My mom died of heart disease at age fifty-five. A few months after she died, my youngest sister—I'm the oldest of four—was watching 20/20 on television and saw two doctors discussing the symptoms of heart disease. Even though she was just twenty-three at the time, she realized she had many of the same issues they were talking about, including dizziness and a really high heart rate. She had heart surgery one year to the day after mom died. Knowing how strong of a hereditary component heart disease has, I became very passionate about educating myself and doing all I could to take care of myself.

I'm not a smoker or drinker, but eating is my weakest link. I have been an emotional eater and yo-yo dieter for as long as I can remember, using food as an emotional crutch. Having lost and gained a ton of weight over the years without dealing with my "real" issues, I always set myself up for failure. Now, and over the past couple of years, I have been working on what the real issues are, making healthier choices, and being more patient and understanding with myself, just like I would be for a friend I care about and love.

I don't cook a lot, so I try to look for healthy choices on restaurant menus. I look up menus online before I go, and when I arrive, I just order what I've already researched. It makes it so much easier.

I've also switched my perspective on eating out. Now I think of it primarily as a time to visit with friends and not as time to sample everything that looks good enough to eat. It's not like it's my last meal!

I also have done my best to get the rest of my life in order and relieve stress. I have taken classes in meditation, I am now a Reiki practitioner, and a couple times a week, I enjoy hot baths. I ensure I always have some quiet time—there is no negotiating there. I am continually learning; I always have a new book or magazine next to my bed. Off and on, I keep a journal; if things are bothering me, I'll write them down.

I have no say over whether I will get the same heart condition as my mother or develop another. I do know I have too much living to do, and I do know that it is up to me—and only me—to take the steps to live a healthier life. I have been working on and making changes in my life in hopes of the chance to live a longer, healthier life. I am choosing to move more, eat healthfully, and take control of my health/weight. I am choosing (with my doctor's advice) to manage my cholesterol and blood pressure and not to ignore symptoms that could possibly mean heart disease. It's a long road and needs to be taken one step at a time.

Buddy Up

One of the keys to the HAPPY Heart program is that everybody participating in it knows that somebody, whether it's a fellow participant or a health coach, has their back. Take time to recruit a trusted friend or family member to be your own health coach; ask that the two of you be in contact, either by phone, email, or in person, at least once a week. "Everybody needs a sounding board," says Traynor, "Somebody who can cheer you on when you're doing well and somebody who isn't afraid to confront and catch you when you're slipping." Similarly, you need to be comfortable and safe enough with this person to be able to call her and say, "I'm really having a tough time: can you help me?" One of the keys of having a health coach or buddy is accountability. If you know someone is going to check and see if you got out of bed and walked three miles in the morning, you are more likely to do it than if nobody is checking in on you.

If you want to make your goals more public, there are plenty of Internet support groups with people who will have the same goals as you do.

Have a Plan

You don't need to be robotic, but you do need to be methodical about your day and your goals. Before you go to bed at night, think about the day ahead. What do you have to do? What food do you have to eat? When will you take time to exercise, meditate, or relax? Expand on that perspective, and you realize you need to be organized and thoughtful to be healthy. You can't eat well if you don't have the right groceries; you can't go for a walk if it's icy outside; you can't stay calm at a heated family dinner if you haven't previously thought about how you are going to behave. But if you shop weekly with a detailed list, have an exercise DVD you can do in bad weather, and collect and center yourself with the relaxation response before heading over to your sister's house, then living in a healthy way doesn't feel like so much of a hassle.

Identify Your Triggers

Another part of the planning process is figuring out when and why you do the things you do. Most unhealthy behaviors are set off by a certain situation: your favorite television show is on, so you get to eat a row of Oreos; you're out with your friends and they smoke socially, so you do too; you get stressed out by your boss at work, so you come home and pick a fight with your spouse. If you're trying to change a certain behavior, change the trigger associated with it: watch your television show at the gym, while you walk on the treadmill; ask your friends not to smoke around you; after you leave work, spend ten minutes immediately going through the Relaxation Response (page 107) so you don't take your job-related stress home with you.

Marcia's Story

I'm sixty-two, and I've had issues with obesity since my twenties; I used to have to call the fire department to help me get up when I fell down in my home. I have a PhD in psychology, yet could not control my brain and stomach connection. I would wake up hungry and go to bed hungry. I was addicted to sugar, starch, and the way that food made me feel.

I've also been on blood pressure medications since my twenties; my father died of a heart attack at age sixty, and he also had issues with blood pressure. Despite being on five blood pressure medications, my blood pressure would on occasion shoot up to 210/150.

I went to see Dr. Wood to see if she had other ideas that might work for my blood pressure; one day, while I was in her office, I saw a gym there and she mentioned there was a program called Learn to Be Lean for men and women. (*Note: This was before HAPPY Heart started.*) That was the beginning of my starting to turn my life around. Every week for three months, a different speaker, like a doctor, nurse, or nutritionist, would speak on some aspect of heart health. Then we'd exercise after every meeting. My heaviest weight was 303 pounds, and I could barely walk on the treadmill, but a nurse was beside me cheering me on and helping me if I needed it.

My assignment was to walk a mile every day, either on the treadmill or outside, for those three months. I hated it. I had never liked walking. I used to get dropped off at the grocery store at the entrance, and then walk slowly with a cart. I never walked anywhere without my walker or other support. But I knew I had to do my daily mile and I never missed a day.

Then I saw a sign at the store for water aerobics at the YMCA. I love to swim. I wondered if I could do that, so I tried. I love it. I love that I have to get out of my house and go. I love the women in the class. I go six times a week and hate it when I look at the clock and see that the class is going to end. I found the place that made me happy.

I changed my eating habits too. I make all my own meals and adhere to a very strict diet. Pretty much every day I eat oatmeal and blueberries for breakfast; homemade chicken soup for lunch; salmon or sardines and steamed veggies for dinner; snacks of hard-boiled eggs, chopped-up chicken, rice cakes with peanut butter.

That may sound really restricted, but it's worked for me. I used to feel sick every day. I never, ever felt good. The word *unhealthy* doesn't even begin to cover it. I took one pill for something, and another for something else, and then the pills would interact, and I'd feel even sicker. I honestly felt like I was at war with my body.

I've gone from taking 40 to 80 mg of five blood pressure medications to 10 mg of one-and-a-half. My BMI has dropped from 49 to 32. My daughter no longer has to tie my shoes for me. I don't have to keep the air conditioning on in the house all year long, even in the dead of winter, so that I can breathe. I don't have to remember my medications when I leave the house. I now weigh 203 pounds.

Although I'd like to get down to 170 pounds, I feel like a functioning human being now. If I want to take a walk, I can. In fact, I can run. I told my daughter the other day that I wanted to run to the end of the hall. I haven't run since I was a little girl. I did it and felt phenomenal. I feel like I can do anything now.

Be Patient

Experts differ on how long you need to do something for it to become a habit; the range goes from eighteen days to six months. Because everybody is different, it is best not to set a time limit on yourself. Instead, try not to judge the process; just tell yourself that you're going to commit to the habit for as long as it takes. The HAPPY Heart patients saw bigger changes in their health during the second year, compared to the first. Yes, that's a long time to wait, but isn't an improved life span and better quality of life worth 365 days or more? "It can be surprising how long it takes to get from point A to point B," admits Culhane-Hermann, "Especially when you want to be at point Z."

Don't Beat Yourself Up for Slipups

As you set out to be smarter at heart, you will have periods of regression and regret. It's human nature. The key when you get off track is to simply let it go. Don't dwell on it, don't think that you've failed, don't discredit all the hard work you've done up to this point. Instead, try to analyze the situation and find the cause of the slipup. When Traynor asks somebody why she went back to smoking and she replies, "Well, my brother died." Traynor pulls apart the situation. "Let's talk about sadness and when you get depressed," she'll suggest, "because there will be more sad times in your life." A person starts smoking again because of sadness and the stress that the sadness brings to her life. "That's when you realize how closely the heart and head are connected," she says, "How you feel affects how you think and how you'll act." Understanding that and having a cigarette substitute in place for when another debilitating event occurs lessens the chance that you'll go for a nicotine fix.

Push Yourself

This final bit of advice might seem incongruent with the more compassionate tips, but the reality is that making a change requires stepping slightly out of your comfort zone. You might feel "off" for a few days, you might lose some friends who don't condone your new behavior, you might mourn the loss of old relationships, you might not like the taste of whole grain bread.

But, as an analogy, keep in mind that the way you build strong muscles is through strength training; when you lift weights, the motion actually makes microscopic tears in your muscles. Over the course of the next few days, the muscles repair themselves and come back stronger and more capable. When you're uncomfortable and, quite frankly, sick of it all, remind yourself that you're tearing down your life's virtual muscles right now. Before you know it, you'll recover and be happier and healthier for it.

Where to go from here? Anywhere—and bonus points if you walk or ride your bike. Seriously, heart disease is the number one killer of women, but it doesn't have to be that way. You now have a handful of tools that can help you take control over your risk for heart disease, as well as other game changers like cancer, diabetes, metabolic syndrome, and many other health maladies.

Do I expect you to swallow this whole book in one gulp? Absolutely not. What I would gently recommend, though, is that you keep it somewhere you'll see it regularly: your bedside table, a coffee table, the backpack you take on the subway to work. Turn to a bridge you feel like needs a little work, and pick out one or two things you can try today. Cook a meal at home; give a relationship some TLC; smile; take some deep breaths; let some light into your world; do whatever it happens to be that you need. I promise you, with some mindful effort to make small changes, you will see bigger and substantial changes sooner than you think.

If you are already living with cardiovascular disease, I need you to remember that it is not a death sentence. With this book—and again, some effort on your part—you have the life-changing power that can help prevent further complications of heart disease. You cannot change the past, but you can certainly build a healthier future for yourself by taking the steps outlined in this book.

I want to end the modification bridge reinforcing how important community is. It's the backbone of HAPPY Heart and my life. Be sure to recognize the people who make up your community: celebrate your victories with them, let them comfort you during trying times, and allow them to support the healthy choices you make in your life.

But I challenge you, as you read and reread this book, to expand your community. As you know, heart disease affects way too many women, and chances are, you're friends with somebody who is either going to be or has been touched by the disease. Invite her along on your journey. Not only will you have a buddy with whom you can comb the aisles of the grocery store as you look for reduced sodium products, but more importantly, the world will have (at least) two more women who are smart at heart.

Three Easy Steps Across the Modification Bridge

1. Identify the areas in your life that need work.
2. Pick the one that feels most conquerable to you right now. Break up your improvement plan into small, doable tasks.
3. Get going!

POSTSCRIPT:
STAYING SMART AT HEART

While I have made enormous positive changes in my life over the past decade, some of which were spurred on by the classic crisis-equals-opportunity mode, I found myself needing a life touch-up in the past six months. During the course of writing this book, my father, a constant presence in my life since my birth and a major source of support for me over the past decade in particular, became quite ill and then passed away. Following his death, difficult family dynamics arose and pitted once loving siblings against one another. All of this happened during the dark, cold days of winter, which made everything even tougher to take. Sad and frustrated, I found myself making excuses not to exercise, sleeping excessively, and coming home every night and pouring myself a glass—or two—of wine. (Look at that: my environment and relationships and my health were all intertwined . . . funny how that works.)

I was so caught up in the family drama, I barely gave myself a chance to fully grieve, let alone begin the healing process. One day I was sitting in my room writing in my journal when it hit me that the best way to honor my father would be to continue down the path he always encouraged me to follow. He knew I was happiest and healthiest when I was totally engaged in my life, embracing my roles as a mother, daughter, doctor, and friend. I recognized that I needed—and wanted—to make a change.

I knew I needed to knock out the unnecessary nocturnal glasses of wine that had become the norm, and in their place, set a realistic goal with a tangible outcome. But nothing was catching my eye, until an opportunity fell into my lap. (Thank you, universe, for watching out for me.) I was offered the opportunity to run the Boston Marathon for Tedy's Team, a nonprofit organization founded by former New England Patriot Tedy Bruschi. Tedy suffered a mild stroke and formed the team to raise money for the American Stroke and American Heart Association. In my mind, this was a win-win situation: a challenging athletic opportunity to get me back on track and a chance to contribute to a cause that was near and dear to my heart. It was a no-brainer. I obviously want to help the professional cardiac associations, and my mother died from complications of a stroke. She actually had the same heart defect that led to the stroke that Tedy had, but fortunately, his was treated early on. And my dear father died of complications of heart failure, so it would be a good way to honor them both.

Armed with motivation I never knew I had, I set out by making a list of the steps I needed to follow to pull it off. First, I had to clean up my diet. I needed to heed the advice of the AHA guidelines and work on eating at least five servings of fresh fruits and vegetables per day. Eating that volume of fresh fruits and veggies left me feeling full and certainly helped diminish my cravings for carbohydrates and empty calories. As serendipity would have it, I managed to bump into a sports nutritionist during a research meeting related to HAPPY Heart. When she found out I was going to be running the marathon, she emailed me some nutritional guidelines. Between her professional advice and that of my sixteen-year-old son, who is a dedicated runner and well read in nutrition, I eliminated trans fats, high fructose corn syrup, and processed foods with nasty ingredients hidden deep within the ingredient list. I started incorporating more whole grains and fresh fruits and vegetables into my diet, and began to eat whole wheat pastas and brown rice, in place of their white and less healthy cousins. I decided to save the wine for the weekend or dinners out with friends.

Then I had to find my exercise mojo—and quick. I had previously run four marathons so I knew I could go the distance, but I really only had seven weeks to train because the Tedy offer came late. (Most runners take at least three months, if not more, to prepare for a marathon.) I would just have to buckle down. Because I had a defined goal within a specific period of time, I focused on a practical and safe training plan: one that would get me across the finish line happy, healthy, and injury free. The winter weather in Boston wasn't exactly ideal for long runs outside, so I focused on becoming fitter indoors, through treadmill running, cycling, indoor rowing, and swimming. As the weather improved, so did the frequency of my long runs on the road—and the quality of my sleep. Thanks to the increased exercise, less alcohol, and a whole lot of motivation, I went from four to five hours of interrupted sleep to eight hours of real rest.

In addition to the more practical changes I made, I also realized that a positive attitude and just showing up day after day count for a lot. My prior marathon—and life—experience taught me that no matter how fast or slow I run, there are going to be moments when I wouldn't feel great. Just keeping my feet headed in the right direction and breathing deeply help the discomfort pass. Before I know it, the second (and third and fourth) winds will hit.

When race day came, I surrounded myself with as many supportive people as I could. A group of friends was waiting for me at the finish line. In my pack around my waist, I carried a picture of my parents—and in my heart, I carried a lifetime of memories. My fifteen-year-old daughter was at mile twenty waiting to run the last 6.2 miles with me, and I was proud to lead by example for her: even though I wasn't feeling great, I kept on putting one foot in front of the other.

On April 18, 2011, aided by a nice tailwind on a perfect running day, I crossed the finish line of the 115th Boston Marathon. Once again, I had set my life back on the path I wanted to be on. My attitude was as sunny as the bright orb in the sky above me, and, as I reveled in my postrace glow, I knew that my dad would have been proud of me for once again taking the reins and embracing my life.

I got over one speed bump and have been once again reintroduced to the path of creating the life I want to lead on a daily basis. I have no doubt that there are further speed bumps down the road waiting for me—and for you. Despite how many times we get thrown off course, we all have the potential to return to the path of health and happiness. I plan on seeing all of you there.

NOTES

Chapter 1

1. L. Mosca et al., "Effectiveness-Based Guidelines for the Prevention of Cardiovascular Disease in Women—2011 Update," *Circulation* 123, no. 11 (2011): 1243.

2. D. Lloyd-Jones et al., "Heart Disease and Stroke Statistics—2010 Update: A Report from the American Heart Association," *Circulation* 121 (2010): e46–e215. National Cancer Institute, "SEER Cancer Statistics Review 1975–2003," available online at http://seer.cancer.gov/csr/1975_2003/results_single/sect_01_table.01.pdf.

3. L. Mosca, "Effectiveness-Based Guidelines," 1243. (See note 1.)

4. Ibid.

5. R. Winslow, "Hearts Actually Can Break," *Wall Street Journal,* February 9, 2010.

6. M. Fiuzat, "United States Stock Market Performance and Acute Myocardial Infarction Rates in 2008–2009 (from the Duke Databank for Cardiovascular Disease)," *American Journal of Cardiology* 106, no. 11 (2010): 1545–49.

7. W. Ma et al., "Stock Volatility as a Risk Factor for Coronary Heart Disease Death," *European Heart Journal* 32, no. 8 (2011): 1006–11.

8. S. S. Anand et al., "INTERHEART Study," *European Heart Journal* 29, no. 7 (2008): 932–40. K. K. Teo et al., "Potentially Modifiable Risk Factors Associated with Myocardial Infarction in China: The INTERHEART China Study," *Heart* 95, no. 22 (2009): 1857–64.

9. M. F. O'Connor et al., "When Grief Heats Up: Pro-Inflammatory Cytokines Predict Regional Brain Activation," *Neuroimage* 47, no. 3 (2009): 891–96.

10. E. Kross et al., "Social Rejection Shares Somatosensory Representations with Physical Pain," *Proceedings of the National Academy of Sciences of the United States of America* 108, no. 15 (2011): 6270–75.

11. J. Sugawara et al., "Effect of Mirthful Laughter on Vascular Function," *American Journal of Cardiology* 106, no. 6 (2010): 856–59.

12. S. Dockray et al., "Positive Affect and Psychobiological Processes," *Neuroscience & Biobehavioral Reviews* 35, no. 1 (2010): 69–75.

13. Y. Chida et al., "Positive Psychological Well-Being and Mortality: A Quantitative Review of Prospective Observational Studies," *Psychosomatic Medicine* 70, no. 7 (2008): 741–56.

14. J. Holt-Lunstad et al., "Social Relationships and Mortality Risk: A Meta-Analytic Review," *PLoS Medicine* 27, no.7 (2010): e1000316.

15. S. G. Post, "Altruism, Happiness, and Health: It's Good to Be Good," *International Journal of Behavioral Medicine* 12, no. 2 (2005): 66–77.

16. Christopher Peterson and Martin Seligman, *Character Strengths and Virtues: A Handbook and Classification* (New York: Oxford University Press, 2004).

17. F. Fujita et al., "Life Satisfaction Set Point: Stability and Change," *Journal of Personality and Social Psychology* 88, no. 1 (2005): 158–64.

18. B. Andersen et al., "Psychological, Behavioral, and Immune Changes After a Psychological Intervention: A Clinical Trial," *Journal of Clinical Oncology* 22, no. 17 (2004): 3570–80.

Chapter 2

1. G. Heiss et al., "Health Risks and Benefits 3 Years After Stopping Randomized Treatment with Estrogen and Progestin," *Journal of the American Medical Association* 299, no. 9 (2008): 1036–45.

2. K. L. Thomas et al., "Racial Differences in Long-Term Survival Among Patients with Coronary Artery Disease," *American Heart Journal* 160, no. 4 (2010): 744–51.

3. Centers for Disease Control and Prevention (CDC), 2011, "U.S. Obesity Trends: Trends by State 1985–2009," available online at www.cdc.gov/obesity/data/trends.html.

4. P. W. Wilson et al., "Overweight and Obesity as Determinants of Cardiovascular Risk: The Framingham Experience," *Archives of Internal Medicine* 162, no. 16 (2002): 1867–72.

5. American Heart Association, 2011, "Smoking: Do You Really Know the Risks?," available online at www.heart.org/HEARTORG/Getting Healthy/QuitSmoking/QuittingSmoking/Smoking-Do-you-really-know-the-risks_UCM_322718_Article.jsp.

6. L. Shahab et al., "Do Ex-Smokers Report Feeling Happier Following Cessation? Evidence from a Cross-Sectional Survey," *Nicotine & Tobacco Research* 11, no. 5 (2009): 553–57.

7. Centers for Disease Control and Prevention (CDC), 2011, "High Blood Pressure Facts," available online at www.cdc.gov/bloodpressure/facts.htm.

8. American Heart Association, 2011, "Understand Your Risk for High Blood Pressure," available online at www.heart.org/HEARTORG/ Conditions/HighBloodPressure/UnderstandYourRiskforHighBlood Pressure/Understand-Your-Risk-for-High-Blood-Pressure_UCM_ 002052_Article.jsp.

9. CDC, 2011, "High Blood Pressure Facts," (see note 7).

10. Center for Science in the Public Interest, 2009, "Heart Attack Entrées and Side Orders of Stroke," available online at www.cspinet.org/new/ 200905111.html.

11. R. Puchades et al., "White-Coat Hypertension in the Elderly, Echocardiographic Analysis, A Substudy of the EPICARDIAN Project," *Revista Española de Cardiología* 63, no. 11 (2010): 1377–81.

12. G. Mancia et al., "Long-Term Risk of Sustained Hypertension in White-Coat or Masked Hypertension," *Hypertension* 54, no. 2 (2009): 226–32.

13. American Heart Association, 2010, "Frequently Asked Questions About Some Common Foods," available online at www.heart.org/ HEARTORG/GettingHealthy/NutritionCenter/HealthyDietGoals/ Frequently-Asked-Questions-About-Some-Common-Foods_UCM_ 316512_Article.jsp.

14. National Diabetes Information Clearinghouse, 2011, "National Diabetes Statistics, 2011," available online at diabetes.niddk.nih.gov/dm/pubs/ statistics/index.htm#fast.

15. Ibid.

16. Ibid.

17. World Socialist Website, 2003, "One-Third of US Children Born in 2000 at Risk for Diabetes," available online at www.wsws.org/articles/ 2003/jun2003/diab-j19.shtml.

18. National Diabetes Information Clearinghouse. "National Diabetes Statistics, 2011."

19. W. C. Knowler et al., "Reduction in the Incidence of Type 2 Diabetes with Lifestyle Intervention or Metformin," *New England Journal of Medicine* 346, no. 6 (2002): 393–403.

20. J. H. O'Keefe et al., "Alcohol and Cardiovascular Health: The Razor-Sharp Double-Edged Sword," *Journal of the American College of Cardiology* 50, no. 11 (2007): 1009–14.

21. M. Schutze et al., "Alcohol Attributable Burden of Incidence of Cancer in Eight European Countries Based on Results from Prospective Cohort Study," *British Medical Journal* 342 (2011): d1584.

22. L. W. Jones et al., "Early Breast Cancer Therapy and Cardiovascular Injury," *Journal of the American College of Cardiology* 50, no. 15 (2007): 1435–41.

Chapter 3

1. J. Dimsdale, "What Does Heart Disease Have to Do with Anxiety?" *Journal of the American College of Cardiology* 51, no. 6 (2010): 47.

2. N. Frasure-Smith et al., "Depression and Myocardial Infarction," *Journal of the American Medical Association* 270, no. 15 (1993): 1819–25.

3. L. D. Kubzansky et al., "The Clinical Impact of Negative Psychological States: Expanding the Spectrum of Risk for Coronary Artery Disease," *Psychosomatic Medicine* 67, Suppl. 1 (2005): S10–14.

4. C. A. Low et al., "Psychosocial Factors in the Development of Heart Disease in Women: Current Research and Future Directions," *Psychosomatic Medicine* 72, no. 9 (2010): 842–54.

5. K. D. László et al., "Anger Expression and Prognosis After a Coronary Event in Women," *International Journal of Cardiology* 140, no. 1 (2010): 60–65.

6. Y. Chida et al., "The Association of Anger and Hostility with Future Coronary Heart Disease: A Meta-Analytic Review of Prospective Evidence," *Journal of the American College of Cardiology* 53, no. 11 (2009): 936–46.

7. World Health Organization, 2010, "Depression," available online at www.who.int/mental_health/management/depression/definition/en/.

8. National Institute of Mental Health, "Major Depressive Disorder Among Adults," available online at www.nimh.nih.gov/statistics/1MDD_ADULT.shtml.

9. V. Vaccarino et al., "Major Depression and Coronary Flow Reserve Detected by Positron Emission Tomography," *Archives of Internal Medicine* 169, no. 18 (2009): 1668–76.

10. W. Whang et al., "Depression and Risk of Sudden Cardiac Death and Coronary Heart Disease in Women: Results from the Nurses' Health Study," *Journal of the American College of Cardiology* 53, no. 11 (2009): 950–58.

11. H. Bohman et al., "Thicker Carotid Intima Layer, Thinner Media Layer, and Higher Intima/Media Ratio in Women with Recurrent Depressive Disorders: A Pilot Study Using Non-invasive High Frequency Ultrasound," *World Journal of Biological Psychiatry* 11, no. 1 (2010): 71–75.

12. H. Nabi et al., "Effects of Depressive Symptoms and Coronary Heart Disease and Their Interactive Associations on Mortality in Middle-Aged Adults: The Whitehall II Cohort Study," *Heart* 96, no. 20 (2010): 1645–50.

13. A. Sherwood et al., "Worsening Depressive Symptoms Are Associated with Adverse Clinical Outcomes in Patients with Heart Failure," *Journal of the American College of Cardiology* 57, no. 4 (2011): 418–23.

14. H. T. May et al., "Depression After Coronary Artery Disease Is Associated with Heart Failure," *Journal of the American College of Cardiology* 53, no. 16 (2009): 1440–47.

15. J. Dimsdale, "What Does Heart Disease Have to Do with Anxiety?" *Journal of the American College of Cardiology* 51, no. 6 (2010): 47.

16. A. M. Roest et al., "Anxiety and Risk of Incident Coronary Heart Disease: A Meta-Analysis," *Journal of the American College of Cardiology* 56, no. 1 (2010): 38–46.

17. B. J. Shen et al., "Anxiety Characteristics Independently and Prospectively Predict Myocardial Infarction in Men: The Unique Contribution of Anxiety Among Psychologic Factors," *Journal of the American College of Cardiology* 51, no. 2 (2008): 113–19.

18. E. Diener et al., "Happy People Live Longer: Subjective Well-Being Contributes to Health and Longevity," *Applied Psychology: Health and Well-Being* 3, no. 1 (2011): 1–43.

19. Science Daily, 2011, "Happiness Improves Health and Lengthens Life, Review Finds," *Science Daily*, available online at www.sciencedaily.com/releases/2011/03/110301122156.htm.

20. S. Cohen et al., "Positive Emotional Style Predicts Resistance to Illness After Experimental Exposure to Rhinovirus or Influenza A Virus," *Psychosomatic Medicine* 68, no. 6 (2006): 809–15.

21. G. Ostir et al., "Associations Between Positive Emotion and Recovery of Functional Status Following Stroke," *Psychosomatic Medicine* 70, no. 4 (2008): 404–9.

22. M. Siahpush et al., "Happiness and Life Satisfaction Prospectively Predict Self-Rated Health, Physical Health, and the Presence of Limiting, Long-Term Health Conditions," *American Journal of Health Promotion* 23, no. 1 (2008): 18–26.

23. D. Blanchflower et al., "Hypertension and Happiness Across Nations," *Journal of Health Economics* 27, no. 2 (2007): 218–233.

24. K. E. Buchanan et al., "Acts of Kindness and Acts of Novelty Affect Life Satisfaction," *Journal of Social Psychology* 150, no. 3 (2010): 235–37.

Chapter 4

1. American Psychological Association, 2011, "How Does Stress Affect Us?," available online at www.apa.org/helpcenter/stress-effects.aspx.

2. American Psychological Association, 2011, "Health and Stress," available online at www.apa.org/news/press/releases/stress/health-stress.aspx.

3. American Psychological Association, 2011, "Gender and Stress," available online at www.apa.org/news/press/releases/stress/gender-stress.aspx.

4. S. Cohen et al., "Who's Stressed? Distributions of Psychological Stress in the United States in Probability Samples from 1983, 2006 and 2009," available online at www.psy.cmu.edu/~scohen/scales.html.

5. Circulation, 2011, Abstract 18520: "Job Strain, Job Insecurity, and Incident Cardiovascular Disease in the Women's Health Study," *Circulation*, available online at http://circ.ahajournals.org/cgi/content/meeting_abstract/122/21_MeetingAbstracts/A18520.

6. K. Orth-Gomér et al., "Marital Stress Worsens Prognosis in Women with Coronary Heart Disease: The Stockholm Female Coronary Risk Study," *Journal of the American Medical Association* 284, no. 23 (2000): 3008–14.

7. E. Epel et al., "Accelerated Telomere Shortening in Response to Life Stress," *Proceedings of the National Academy of Science of the United States of America* 101, no. 49 (2004): 17312–15.

8. V. E. Burns et al., "Stress, Coping, and Hepatitis B Antibody Status," *Psychosomatic Medicine* 64, no. 2 (2002): 287–93. R. Glaser et al., "Chronic Stress Modulates the Immune Response to a Pneumococcal Pneumonia Vaccine," *Psychosomatic Medicine* 62, no. 6 (2000): 804–7.

9. J. K. Kiecolt-Glaser et al., "Chronic Stress and Age-Related Increases in the Proinflammatory Cytokine IL-6," *Proceedings of the National Academy of Science of the United States of America* 100, no. 15 (2003): 9090–5.

10. I. Chiodini et al., "Bone Mineral Density, Prevalence of Vertebral Fractures, and Bone Quality in Patients with Adrenal Incidentalomas With and Without Subclinical Hypercortisolism: An Italian Multicenter Study," *Journal of Clinical Endocrinology & Metabolism* 94, no. 9 (2009): 3207–14.

11. R. Peled et al., "Breast Cancer, Psychological Distress, and Life Events Among Young Women," *BMC Cancer* 8 (2008): 245.

12. C. A. Shively et al., "Social Stress, Visceral Obesity, and Coronary Artery Atherosclerosis in Female Primates," *Obesity (Silver Spring)* 17, no. 8 (2009): 1513–20.

13. J. P. Block et al., "Psychosocial Stress and Change in Weight Among US Adults," *American Journal of Epidemiology* 170, no. 2 (2009): 181–92.

14. L. V. Doering et al., "A Literature Review of Depression, Anxiety, and Cardiovascular Disease in Women," *Journal of Obstetric, Gynecologic, & Neonatal Nursing* 40, no. 3 (2011): 348–61.

15. M. A. Miller et al., "Gender Differences in the Cross-Sectional Relationships Between Sleep Duration and Markers of Inflammation: Whitehall II Study," *Sleep* 32, no. 7 (2009): 857–64.

16. A. V. Nedeltcheva et al., "Insufficient Sleep Undermines Dietary Efforts to Reduce Adiposity," *Annals of Internal Medicine* 153, no. 7 (2010): 435–41.

17. Herbert Benson, *The Relaxation Response* (New York: HarperTorch, 1976).

18. E. E. Hill et al., "Exercise and Circulating Cortisol Levels: The Intensity Threshold Effect," *Journal of Endocrinological Investigation* 31, no. 7 (2008): 587–91.

19. M. Ehud et al., "Here and Now: Yoga in Israeli Schools," *International Journal of Yoga* 3, no. 2 (2010): 42–47.

20. J. A. Häusser et al., "Endocrinological and Psychological Responses to Job Stressors: An Experimental Test of the Job Demand-Control Model," *Psychoneuroendocrinology*. Jan 20, 2011 [Epub ahead of print].

21. L. L. Jefferson, "Exploring Effects of Therapeutic Massage and Patient Teaching in the Practice of Diaphragmatic Breathing on Blood Pressure, Stress, and Anxiety in Hypertensive African-American Women: An Intervention Study," *Journal of National Black Nurses' Association* 21, no. 1 (2010): 17–24.

22. W. Zhou et al., "Review of Trials Examining the Use of Acupuncture to Treat Hypertension," *Future Cardiology* 2, no. 3 (2006): 287–92. J. Hervik et al., "Quality of Life of Breast Cancer Patients Medicated with Anti-Estrogens, 2 Years After Acupuncture Treatment: A Qualitative Study," *International Journal of Women's Health* 2 (2010): 319–25.

Chapter 5

1. J. Van der Steeg et al., "Obesity Affects Spontaneous Pregnancy Chances in Subfertile, Ovulatory Women," *Human Reproduction Advanced Access* 23, no. 2 (2008): 324–28. F. C. Denison et al., "Increased Maternal BMI Is Associated with an Increased Risk of Minor Complications During Pregnancy with Consequent Cost Implications," *British Journal of Obstetrics and Gynaecology* 116, no. 11 (2009): 1467–72.

2. U.S. Department of Health and Human Services, 2008, "Physical Activity Guidelines for Americans," available online at www.health.gov/PAGuidelines/committeereport.aspx.

3. Ibid.

4. A. Baggish et al., "Training-Specific Changes in Cardiac Structure and Function: A Prospective and Longitudinal Assessment of Competitive Athletes," *Journal of Applied Physiology* 104, no. 4 (2008): 1121–28.

5. J. Cook et al., "Arterial Compliance of Rowers: Implications for Combined Aerobic and Strength Training on Arterial Elasticity," *American Journal of Physiology: Heart and Circulatory Physiology* 290, no. 4 (2006): H1596–600.

6. A. Arbab-Zadeh et al., "Effect of Aging and Physical Activity on Left Ventricular Compliance," *Circulation* 110, no. 13 (2004): 1799–805.

7. R. Gary, "Exercise Self-Efficacy in Older Women with Diastolic Heart Failure: Results of a Walking Program and Education Intervention," *Journal of Gerontological Nursing* 32, no. 7 (2006): 31–39.

8. S. Tolomio et al., "The Effect of a Multicomponent Dual-Modality Exercise Program Targeting Osteoporosis on Bone Health Status and Physical Function Capacity of Postmenopausal Women," *Journal of Women & Aging* 22, no. 4 (2010): 241–54.

9. K. Flack et al., "Aging, Resistance Training, and Diabetes Prevention," *Journal of Aging Research* (2011): 127315.

10. B. Sañudo et al., "Aerobic Exercise Versus Combined Exercise Therapy in Women with Fibromyalgia Syndrome: A Randomized Controlled Trial," *Archives of Physical Medicine and Rehabilitation* 91, no. 12 (2010): 1838–43. K. Mannerkorpi et al., "Does Moderate-to-High Intensity Nordic Walking Improve Functional Capacity and Pain in Fibromyalgia? A Prospective Randomized Controlled Trial," *Arthritis Research & Therapy* 12, no. 5 (2010): R189.

11. B. Lynch et al., "Physical Activity and Breast Cancer Prevention," *Recent Results in Cancer Research* 186, no. 1 (2011): 13–42.

12. A. Y. Arikawa, "Sixteen Weeks of Exercise Reduces C-Reactive Protein Levels in Young Women," *Medicine & Science in Sports & Exercise* 43, no. 6 (2010): 1002–9.

13. K. J. Reid, "Aerobic Exercise Improves Self-Reported Sleep and Quality of Life in Older Adults with Insomnia," *Sleep Medicine* 11, no. 9 (2010): 934–40.

14. R. V. Milani et al., "Reducing Psychosocial Stress: A Novel Mechanism of Improving Survival from Exercise Training," *American Journal of Medicine* 122, no. 10 (2009): 931–38.

15. M. P. Herrin et al., "The Effect of Exercise Training on Anxiety Symptoms Among Patients: A Systematic Review," *Archives of Internal Medicine* 170, no. 4 (2010): 321–31.

16. B. M. Hoffman et al., "Exercise and Pharmacotherapy in Patients with Major Depression: One-Year Follow-Up of the SMILE Study," *Psychosomatic Medicine* 73, no. 2 (2010): 127–33.

17. C. C. Streeter et al., "Yoga Asana Sessions Increase Brain GABA Levels: A Pilot Study," *Journal of Alternative and Complementary Medicine* 13, no. 4 (2007): 419–26.

18. T. Liu-Ambrose et al., "Resistance Training and Executive Functions: A 12-Month Randomized Controlled Trial," *Archives of Internal Medicine* 170, no. 2 (2010): 170–78.

19. U.S. Department of Health and Human Services, 2008, "Physical Activity Guidelines for Americans," available online at www.health.gov/PAGuidelines/committeereport.aspx.

20. Ibid.

21. A. Zutz et al., "Utilization of the Internet to Deliver Cardiac Rehabilitation at a Distance: A Pilot Study," *Telemedicine and e-Health* 13, no. 3 (2007): 323–30.

22. American Congress of Obstetricians and Gynecologists, 2003, "Exercise During Pregnancy," available online at www.acog.org/publications/patient_education/bp119.cfm.

23. K. Goel et al., "Combined Effect of Cardiorespiratory Fitness and Adiposity on Mortality in Patients with Coronary Artery Disease," *American Heart Journal* 161, no. 3 (2010): 590–97.

24. A. Marcus, 2011, "Obese with Strong Heart Beats Thin and Weak," *Reuters Health* March 31, 2011.

25. Centers for Disease Control and Prevention (CDC), 2009, "Body Measurements," available online at www.cdc.gov/nchs/fastats/bodymeas.htm.

26. D. Peterson, 2009, "Music Benefits Exercise, Studies Show," *LiveScience,* available online at www.livescience.com/5799-music-benefits-exercise-studies-show.html.

Chapter 6

1. American Psychological Association, 2008, "Stress in America Annual Report: APA Poll Finds Women Bear Brunt of Nation's Stress, Financial Downturn," available online at www.apa.org/news/press/releases/2008/10/stress-women.aspx.

2. R. T. Mikolajczyk et al., "Food Consumption Frequency and Perceived Stress and Depressive Symptoms Among Students in Three European Countries," *Nutrition Journal* 8 (2009): 31.

3. D. Zellner et al., "Food Selection Changes Under Stress," *Physiology & Behavior* 87 (2006): 789–93.

4. F. B. Hu et al., "Television Watching and Other Sedentary Behaviors in Relation to Risk of Obesity and Type 2 Diabetes Mellitus in Women," *Journal of the American Medical Association* 289, no. 14 (2003): 1785–91.

5. E. Stamatakis et al., "Screen-Based Entertainment Time, All-Cause Mortality, and Cardiovascular Events: Population-Based Study with Ongoing Mortality and Hospital Events Follow-Up," *Journal of the American College of Cardiology* 57, no. 3 (2011): 292–99.

6. L. Mosca, "Effectiveness-Based Guidelines," 1243. (See chapter 1, note 1.)

7. B. Wansink et al., "Shape of Glass and Amount of Alcohol Poured: Comparative Study of Effect of Practice and Concentration," *British Medical Journal* 331, no. 7531 (2005): 1512–14.

8. United States Department of Agriculture, 2011, "Dietary Guidelines for Americans," available online at www.cnpp.usda.gov/dietaryguidelines.htm.

9. American Heart Association, 2011, "American Heart Association Supports New USDA/HHS Dietary Guidelines and Encourages Adherence," available online at www.newsroom.heart.org/index .php?s=43&item=1243.

10. M. Ashwell, "An Examination of the Relationship Between Breakfast, Weight, and Shape," *British Journal of Nursing* 19, no. 18 (2010): 1155–59.

11. Ibid.

12. R. E. Oldham-Cooper et al., "Playing a Computer Game During Lunch Affects Fullness, Memory for Lunch, and Later Snack Intake," *American Journal of Clinical Nutrition* 93, no. 2 (2011): 308–13.

13. P. L. Lutsey et al., "Dietary Intake and the Development of the Metabolic Syndrome: The Atherosclerosis Risk in Communities Study," *Circulation* 117, no. 6 (2008): 754–61.

14. E. D. Shade et al., "Frequent Intentional Weight Loss Is Associated with Lower Natural Killer Cell Cytotoxicity in Postmenopausal Women: Possible Long-Term Immune Effects," *Journal of the American Dietetic Association* 104, no. 6 (2004): 903–12.

15. K. J. Streit et al., "Food Records: A Predictor and Modifier of Weight Change in a Long-Term Weight Loss Program," *Journal of the American Dietetic Association* 91, no. 2 (1991): 213–16.

16. M. J. Wood et al., "Use of Complementary and Alternative Medical Therapies in Patients with Cardiovascular Disease," *American Heart Journal* 145, no. 5 (2003): 806–12.

17. Northwestern University, 2011, "Load Up on Fiber Now, Avoid Heart Disease Later," available online at www.northwestern.edu/newscenter/ stories/2011/03/fiber-heart-disease.html.

Chapter 7

1. J. Holt-Lunstad, "Social Relationships and Mortality Risk." (See chapter 1, note 14.)

2. J. H. Fowler et al., "Dynamic Spread of Happiness in a Large Social Network: Longitudinal Analysis over 20 Years in the Framingham Heart Study," *British Medical Journal* 337 (2008): a2338.

3. L. M. Everett-Haynes, 2010, "Loneliness, Poor Health Appear to Be Linked," *UANews*, University of Arizona, available online at www.uanews.org/printview/32366.

4. A. Steptoe et al., "Loneliness and Neuroendocrine, Cardiovascular, and Inflammatory Stress Responses in Middle-Aged Men and Women," *Psychoneuroendocrinology* 29, no. 5 (2004): 593–611.

5. L. C. Hawkley et al., "Loneliness Predicts Increased Blood Pressure: 5-Year Cross-Lagged Analyses in Middle-Aged and Older Adults," *Psychology and Aging* 25, no. 1 (2010): 132–41.

6. UCLA Health System, 2011, "Loneliness Triggers Unhealthy Immune Response, Study Finds," available online at www.uclahealth.org/body.cfm?id=561&action=detail&ref=1594.

7. Science Daily, 2007, "Loneliness Is a Molecule," *Science Daily*, available online at www.sciencedaily.com/releases2007/09/070913081048.htm.

8. C. Segrin et al., "Functions of Loneliness, Social Support, Health Behaviors, and Stress in Association with Poor Health," *Health Communications* 25, no. 4 (2010): 312–22.

9. S. K. Kumanyika et al., "Trial of Family and Friend Support for Weight Loss in African-American Adults," *Archives of Internal Medicine* 169, no. 19 (2009): 1795–804.

10. J. N. Rosenquist et al., "The Spread of Alcohol Consumption Behavior in a Large Social Network," *Annals of Internal Medicine* 152, no. 7 (2010): 426–33.

11. N. A. Christakis et al., "The Spread of Obesity in a Large Social Network over 32 Years," *New England Journal of Medicine* 357, no. 4 (2007): 370–79.

12. Nicholas A. Christakas and James A. Fowler, *Connected: The Surprising Power of Our Social Networks and How They Shape Our Lives* (New York: Little, Brown and Company, 2008).

13. A. J. O'Malley et al., "Longitudinal Analysis of Large Social Networks: Estimating the Effect of Health Traits on Changes in Friendship Ties," *Statistics in Medicine* 30, no. 9 (2011): 950–64.

14. J. H. Fowler et al., "Correlated Genotypes in Friendship Networks," *Proceedings of the National Academy of Sciences* 108, no. 5 (2011): 1993–97.

15. J. Holt-Lunstad et al., "On the Importance of Relationship Quality: The Impact of Ambivalence in Friendships on Cardiovascular Functioning," *Annals of Behavioral Medicine* 33, no. 3 (2007): 278–90.

16. D. Uno, "Relationship Quality Moderates the Effect of Social Support Given by Close Friends on Cardiovascular Reactivity in Women," *International Journal of Behavioral Medicine* 9, no. 3 (2002): 243–62.

17. U.S. Department of Health and Human Services, 2007, "The Effects of Marriage on Health: A Synthesis of Recent Research Evidence," available online at http://aspe.hhs.gov/hsp/07/marriageonhealth/rb.htm.

18. Ibid.

19. Z. Zhang et al., "Gender, the Marital Life Course, and Cardiovascular Disease in Late Midlife," *Journal of Marriage and Family* 68, no. 3 (2006): 639–57.

20. R. Kaplan et al., "Marital Status and Longevity in the U.S. Population," *Journal of Epidemiology and Community Health* 60, no. 9 (2006): 760–65.

21. M. E. Hughes et al., "Marital Biography and Health at Mid-Life," *Journal of Health and Social Behavior* 50, no. 3 (2009): 344–58.

22. Reuters Health, 2009, "Lasting Marriage Linked to Better Health," available online at www.reuters.com/article/2009/07/27/us-lasting-marriage-idUSTRE56Q4OI20090727.

23. J. K. Kiecolt-Glaser et al., "Hostile Marital Interactions, Proinflammatory Cytokine Production, and Wound Healing," *Archives of General Psychiatry* 62, no. 12 (2005): 1377–84.

24. G. Vince, 2005, "Arguments Dramatically Slow Wound Healing," *New Scientist*, available online at www.newscientist.com/article/dn8418-arguments-dramatically-slow-wound-healing.html.

25. T. W. Smith et al., "Conflict and Collaboration in Middle-Aged and Older Couples: I. Age Differences in Agency and Communion During Marital Interaction," *Psychology and Aging* 24, no. 2 (2009): 259–73.

26. T. W. Smith et al., "Affiliation and Control During Marital Disagreement, History of Divorce, and Asymptomatic Coronary Artery Calcification in Older Couples," *Psychosomatic Medicine* 73, no. 4 (2011): 350–57.

27. W. M. Troxel et al., "Marital Happiness and Sleep Disturbances in a Multi-Ethnic Sample of Middle-Aged Women," *Behavioral Sleep Medicine* 7, no. 1 (2009): 2–19.

28. W. M. Troxel et al., "Marital/Cohabitation Status and History in Relation to Sleep in Midlife Women," *Sleep* 33, no. 7 (2010): 973–81.

29. M. J. Rohrbaugh et al., "Effect of Marital Quality on Eight-Year Survival of Patients with Heart Failure," *American Journal of Cardiology* 98, no. 8 (2006): 1069–72.

30. J. A. Coan et al., "Lending a Hand: Social Regulation of the Neural Response to Threat," *Psychological Science* 17, no. 12 (2006): 1032–9.

31. MSN, 2007, "Stressed Out? Grab Hubby's Hand," available online at http://health.msn.com/womens-health/articlepage.aspx?cp-documentid= 100150881&gt1=8816.

32. G. Keillor, 2006, "That Thing Called Love," *Chicago Tribune*, April 12, 2006.

Chapter 8

1. Breast Cancer.org, 2011, "U.S. Breast Cancer Statistics," available online at www.breastcancer.org/symptoms/understand_bc/statistics.jsp.

2. Christiane Northrup, *Women's Bodies, Women's Wisdom* (New York: Hay House, 2010).

3. G. Ostir et al., "Onset of Frailty in Older Adults and the Protective Role of Positive Affect," *Psychology and Aging* 19, no. 3 (2004): 402–8.

4. D. Danner et al., "Positive Emotions in Early Life and Longevity: Findings from the Nun Study," *Journal of Personality and Social Psychology* 80, no. 5 (2001): 804–813.

5. A. L. Stanton et al., "Randomized, Controlled Trial of Written Emotional Expression and Benefit Finding in Breast Cancer Patients," *Journal of Clinical Oncology* 20, no. 20 (2002): 4160–68.

6. K. B. Zolnierek et al., "Physician Communication and Patient Adherence to Treatment: A Meta-Analysis," *Medical Care* 47, no. 8 (2009): 826–34.

7. J. J. Van Berkum et al., "The Neural Integration of Speaker and Message," *Journal of Cognitive Neuroscience* 20, no. 4 (2008): 580–91.

8. M. R. Mehl et al., "Eavesdropping on Happiness: Well-Being Is Related to Having Less Small Talk and More Substantive Conversations," *Psychological Science* 21, no. 4 (2010): 539–41.

9. R. C. Rabin, 2010, *New York Times* "Well" blog: "Talk Deeply, Be Happy?," available online at http://well.blogs.nytimes.com/2010/03/17/talk-deeply-be-happy/.

10. J. Kruger et al., "Egocentrism over E-mail: Can We Communicate as Well as We Think?" *Journal of Personality and Social Psychology* 89, no. 6 (2005): 925–36.

11. C. Naquin et al., "E-mail Communication and Group Cooperation in Mixed Motive Contexts," *Social Justice Research* 21, no. 4 (2008): 470–89.

12. K. Bessiere et al., "Effects of Internet Use on Health and Depression: A Longitudinal Study," *Journal of Medical Internet Research* 12, no. 1 (2010): e6.

13. UChicago News, 2008, "Breast Cancer in Black Women May Be Connected to Neighborhood Conditions," *UChicago News*, available online at http://news.uchicago.edu/article/2008/03/14/breast-cancer-black-women-may-be-connected-neighborhood-conditions.

14. M. Hertenstein et al., "Smile Intensity in Photographs Predicts Divorce Later in Life," *Motivation and Emotion* 33, no. 2 (2009): 99–105.

15. E. L. Abel et al., "Smile Intensity in Photographs Predicts Longevity," *Psychological Science* 21, no. 4 (2010): 542–44.

16. A. Mehrabian et al., "Inference of Attitudes from Nonverbal Communication in Two Channels," *Journal of Consulting Psychology* 31, no. 3 (1967): 248–58.

17. M. E. Teixeria et al., "Obesity Stigma: A Newly Recognized Barrier to Comprehensive and Effective Type 2 Diabetes Management," *Journal of the American Academy of Nurse Practitioners* 22, no. 10 (2010): 527–33.

18. R. W. Greene, "Lives in the Balance: What Is Collaborative Problem Solving?," available online at www.livesinthebalance.org/what-is-collaborative-problem-solving-cps.

19. BBC News, April 22, 2005, "'Infomania' Worse Than Marijuana," available online at http://news.bbc.co.uk/2/hi/uk_news/4471607.stm.

Chapter 9

1. T. Nawrot et al., "Public Health Importance of Triggers of Myocardial Infarction: A Comparative Risk Assessment," *The Lancet* 377 (2011): 732–40.

2. R. Brook et al., "AHA Scientific Statement: Air Pollution and Cardiovascular Disease," *Circulation* 109 (2004): 2655–71.

3. United States Environmental Protection Agency, "The Inside Story: A Guide to Indoor Air Quality," available online at www.epa.gov/iaq/pubs/insidestory.html.

4. S. A. Glantz et al., "Passive Smoking and Heart Disease, Epidemiology, Physiology, and Biochemistry," *Circulation* 83, no. 1 (1991): 1–12.

5. K. M. Wilson et al., "Tobacco-Smoke Exposure in Children Who Live in Multiunit Housing," *Pediatrics* 127, no. 1 (2011): 85–92.

6. N. Mills et al., "Diesel Exhaust Inhalation Causes Vascular Dysfunction and Impaired Endogenous Fibrinolysis," *Circulation* 112, no. 25 (2005): 3930–36. B. Hoffman et al., "Residential Exposure to Traffic Is Associated with Coronary Atherosclerosis," *Circulation* 116, no. 5 (2007): 489–96.

7. R. Brook, "AHA Scientific Statement: Air Pollution and Cardiovascular Disease," *Circulation* 109 (2004): 2655–2671.

8. S. Mitrione, "Therapeutic Responses to Natural Environments: Using Gardens to Improve Health Care," *Minnesota Medicine* 91, no. 3 (2008): 31–34.

9. D. Yank et al., "Screening Indoor Plants for Volatile Organic Pollutant Removal Efficiency," *HortScience* 44 (2009):1377–81.

10. S. T. Kent et al., "Effect of Sunlight Exposure on Cognitive Function Among Depressed and Non-Depressed Participants: A REGARDS Cross-Sectional Study," *Environmental Health* 8 (2009): 34.

11. Heschong Mahone Group, "Daylighting and Productivity," available online at www.h-m-g.com/projects/daylighting/projects-pier.htm.

12. M. Hamer et al., "Dose-Response Relationship Between Physical Activity and Mental Health: The Scottish Health Survey," *British Journal of Sports Medicine* 43, no. 14 (2009): 1111–14.

13. R. W. Allen et al., "An Air Filter Intervention Study of Endothelial Function Among Healthy Adults in a Woodsmoke-Impacted Community," *American Journal of Respiratory and Critical Care Medicine* 183, no. 9 (2011): 1222–30.

14. Office of Dietary Supplements: National Institutes of Health, "Dietary Supplement Fact Sheet: Vitamin D," available online at http://ods.od.nih.gov/factsheets/vitamind.

15. Environmental Working Group, 2011, "Shopper's Guide to Pesticides in Produce," available online at www.ewg.org/foodnews/summary/.

16. Cindy Glovinsky, *One Thing at a Time: 100 Simple Ways to Live Clutter-Free Every Day* (New York: St. Martin's Griffin, 2004).

Chapter 10

1. J. Schneider et al., "Effects of Stress Reduction on Clinical Events in African Americans with Coronary Heart Disease: A Randomized Controlled Trial," *Circulation* 120 (2009): S461.

2. B. K. Hölzel et al., "Mindfulness Practice Leads to Increases in Regional Brain Gray Matter Density," *Psychiatry Research: Neuroimaging* 191, no. 1 (2011): 36–43.

3. Massachusetts General Hospital, 2011, "Mindfulness Meditation Changes Brain Structure in 8 Weeks," available online at www.massgeneral.org/about/pressrelease.aspx?id=1329.

4. L. Bernardi et al., "Effect of Rosary Prayer and Yoga Mantras on Autonomic Cardiovascular Rhythms: Comparative Study," *British Medical Journal* 323, no. 7237 (2001): 1446–49.

5. J. Bradt et al., "Music for Stress and Anxiety Reduction in Coronary Heart Disease Patients," *Cochrane Database of Systematic Reviews* 2 (2009): CD006577.

6. H. J. Trappe, "The Effects of Music on the Cardiovascular System and Cardiovascular Health," *Heart* 96, no. 23 (2010): 1868–71.

7. L. Bernardi et al., "Cardiovascular, Cerebrovascular, and Respiratory Changes Induced by Different Types of Music in Musicians and Non-Musicians: The Importance of Silence," *Heart* 92, no. 4 (2006): 445–52.

8. American Heart Association, "European Perspectives," *Circulation* 116 (2007): F139–F144.

9. K. Geue et al., "An Overview of Art Therapy Interventions for Cancer Patients and the Results of Research," *Complementary Therapies in Medicine* 18, no. 3–4 (2010): 160–70.

10. B. S. Thomley et al., "Effects of a Brief, Comprehensive, Yoga-Based Program on Quality of Life and Biometric Measures in an Employee Population: A Pilot Study," *Explore (NY)* 7, no. 1 (2011): 27–29.

11. J. W. Carson et al., "A Pilot Randomized Controlled Trial of the Yoga of Awareness Program in the Management of Fibromyalgia," *Pain* 151, no. 2 (2010): 530–39.

12. R. Garrett et al., 2011, "Becoming Connected: The Lived Experience of Yoga Participation after Stroke," *Disability and Rehabilitation*, April 21 [Epub ahead of print].

13. G. Y. Yeh et al., "Effects of Tai Chi Mind-Body Movement Therapy on Functional Status and Exercise Capacity in Patients with Chronic Heart Failure: A Randomized Controlled Trial," *American Journal of Medicine* 117, no. 8 (2004): 541–48.

14. G. Y. Yeh et al., "Tai Chi Exercise in Patients with Chronic Heart Failure: A Randomized Clinical Trial," *Archives of Internal Medicine* 171, no. 8 (2011): 750–57.

ABOUT THE AUTHORS

Malissa Wood, MD, is the co-director of the Corrigan Women's Heart Health Program at Massachusetts General Hospital. She sits on the board of the Northeast affiliate of the American Heart Association, and she has appeared on the *Today* show for a national Go Red public service announcement. She lives with her family in Boston, Massachusetts.

Dimity McDowell, a health and fitness writer, has been a contributing editor at *Shape*, *Sports Illustrated Women*, and *Women's Health*. Her writing has appeared in the *New York Times*, *Real Simple*, and *Runner's World*, among others. She is the coauthor of *Run Like a Mother* and *Train Like a Mother*. She lives with her family in Denver, Colorado.

INDEX